Sjogren's Disease

Editor

R. HAL SCOFIELD

RHEUMATIC DISEASE CLINICS OF NORTH AMERICA

www.rheumatic.theclinics.com

Consulting Editor
MICHAEL H. WEISMAN

August 2016 • Volume 42 • Number 3

ELSEVIER

1600 John F. Kennedy Boulevard • Suite 1800 • Philadelphia, Pennsylvania, 19103-2899
http://www.theclinics.com

RHEUMATIC DISEASE CLINICS OF NORTH AMERICA Volume 42, Number 3

August 2016 ISSN 0889-857X, ISBN 13: 978-0-323-45987-7

Editor: Jennifer Flynn-Briggs
Developmental Editor: Casey Jackson

Rheumatic Disease Clinics of North America (ISSN 0889-857X) is published quarterly by Elsevier Inc., 360 Park Avenue South, New York, NY 10010-1710. Months of issue are February, May, August, and November. Business and editorial offices: 1600 John F. Kennedy Boulevard, Suite 1000, Philadelphia PA 19103-2899. Periodicals postage paid at New York, NY and additional mailing offices. Subscription prices are USD 335.00 per year for US individuals, USD 634.00 per year for US institutions, USD 100.00 per year for US students and residents, USD 395.00 per year for Canadian individuals, USD 791.00 per year for Canadian institutions, USD 465.00 per year for international individuals, USD 791.00 per year for international institutions, and USD 230.00 per year for Canadian and foreign students/residents. To receive student/resident rate, orders must be accompanied by name of affiliated institution, date of term, and the *signature* of program/residency coordinator on institution letterhead. Orders will be billed at individual rate until proof of status received. Foreign air speed delivery is included in all *Clinics* subscription prices. All prices are subject to change without notice. **POSTMASTER:** Send address changes to *Rheumatic Disease Clinics of North America,* Elsevier Health Sciences Division, Subscription Customer Service, 3251 Riverport Lane, Maryland Heights, MO 63043. **Customer Service: 1-800-654-2452 (US and Canada). From outside of the US and Canada: 314-447-8871. Fax: 314-447-8029. For print support, e-mail: JournalsCustomerService-usa@elsevier.com. For online support, e-mail: JournalsOnline Support-usa@elsevier.com.**

Reprints. For copies of 100 or more of articles in this publication, please contact the Commercial Reprints Department, Elsevier Inc., 360 Park Avenue South, New York, New York, 10010-1710; Tel.: +1-212-633-3874, Fax: +1-212-633-3820, and E-mail: reprints@elsevier.com.

Rheumatic Disease Clinics of North America is covered in *MEDLINE/PubMed (Index Medicus), Current Contents/Clinical Medicine, Science Citation Index, ISI/BIOMED,* and *EMBASE/Excerpta Medica.*

Contributors

CONSULTING EDITOR

MICHAEL H. WEISMAN, MD
Cedars-Sinai Chair in Rheumatology, Director, Division of Rheumatology, Professor of
Medicine, Cedars-Sinai Medical Center, Distinguished Professor, David Geffen School of
Medicine at UCLA, Los Angeles, California

EDITOR

R. HAL SCOFIELD, MD, FACR
Professor, Department of Medicine, College of Medicine, University of Oklahoma
Health Sciences Center; Member, Arthritis and Clinical Immunology Program,
Oklahoma Medical Research Foundation; Staff Physician, Medical Service,
Oklahoma City Department of Veterans Affairs Medical Center, Oklahoma City,
Oklahoma

AUTHORS

JUAN-MANUEL ANAYA, MD, PhD
Center for Autoimmune Diseases Research (CREA), School of Medicine and Health
Sciences, Universidad del Rosario, Bogotá, Colombia

MAURICIO ARCOS-BURGOS, MD, PhD
Genomics and Predictive Medicine, Genome Biology Department, John Curtin School of
Medical Research, ANU College of Medicine, Biology and Environment, The Australian
National University, Canberra, Australia

CHIARA BALDINI, MD, PhD
Rheumatology Unit, University of Pisa, Pisa, Italy

FRANCESCA BARONE, MD, PhD
Research Laboratories, Consultant Rheumatologist, Centre for Translational Inflammation
Research, School of Immunity and Infection, College of Medical and Dental Sciences,
Queen Elizabeth Hospital, Birmingham, United Kingdom

HENDRIKA BOOTSMA, MD, PhD
Professor and Chairman, Department of Rheumatology and Clinical Immunology,
University of Groningen, University Medical Center Groningen, Groningen,
The Netherlands

MICHAEL T. BRENNAN, DDS, MHS
Professor and Chair, Department of Oral Medicine, Carolinas Medical Center, Charlotte,
North Carolina

JOANA CAMPOS, PhD
Centre for Translational Inflammation Research, School of Immunity and Infection,
University of Birmingham, Birmingham, United Kingdom

STEVEN E. CARSONS, MD, FACR
Chief, Division of Rheumatology, Allergy and Immunology, Winthrop University Hospital; Campus Professor of Medicine, Stony Brook University School of Medicine, Stony Brook, Mineola, New York

DIVI CORNEC, MD, PhD
Department of Rheumatology, CHRU Brest; EA 2216, INSERM ESPRI, ERI29, Université de Brest, LabEx IGO, Brest, France

TROY E. DANIELS, DDS, MS
Professor of Oral Medicine and Pathology, Department of Orofacial Sciences, UCSF Schools of Dentistry and Medicine, San Francisco, California

ANUM FAYYAZ, MBBS
Arthritis and Clinical Immunology Program, Oklahoma Medical Research Foundation; Department of Medicine, College of Medicine, University of Oklahoma Health Sciences Center; Medical and Research Services, US Department of Veterans Affairs Hospital, Oklahoma City, Oklahoma

S. LANCE FORSTOT, MD, FACS
Corneal Consultants of Colorado, Littleton, Colorado

GARY FOULKS, MD, FACS
Department of Ophthalmology and Vision Science, University of Louisville School of Medicine, Louisville, Kentucky

CARLA M. FOX, RN
Rheumatology Clinic, Scripps Memorial Hospital, XiMED Medical Group, La Jolla, California

ROBERT I. FOX, MD, PhD
Chief, Rheumatology Clinic, Department of Medicine, Scripps Memorial Hospital, XiMED Medical Group, La Jolla, California

ERLIN HAACKE, MD
Research Fellow, Department of Rheumatology and Clinical Immunology; Department of Pathology and Medical Biology, University of Groningen, University Medical Center Groningen, Groningen, The Netherlands

KATHERINE M. HAMMITT, MA
Sjögren's Syndrome Foundation, Bethesda, Maryland

MAARTEN R. HILLEN, PhD
Centre for Translational Inflammation Research, School of Immunity and Infection, University of Birmingham, Birmingham, United Kingdom; Laboratory of Translational Immunology, University Medical Centre Utrecht, Utrecht, The Netherlands

MALIN V. JONSSON, DMD, PhD
Section for Oral and Maxillofacial Radiology, Department of Clinical Dentistry, Faculty of Medicine and Dentistry, University of Bergen; Broegelmann Research Laboratory, Department of Clinical Medicine, Faculty of Medicine and Dentistry, University of Bergen, Bergen, Norway

STERGIOS KATSIOUGIANNIS, PhD
Assistant Project Scientist, Center for Oral/Head and Neck Oncology Research, School of Dentistry, UCLA, Los Angeles, California

FRANS G.M. KROESE, PhD
Professor, Department of Rheumatology and Clinical Immunology, University of Groningen, University Medical Center Groningen, Groningen, The Netherlands

BIJI T. KURIEN, PhD
Arthritis and Clinical Immunology Program, Oklahoma Medical Research Foundation; Department of Medicine, College of Medicine, University of Oklahoma Health Sciences Center; Medical and Research Services, US Department of Veterans Affairs Hospital, Oklahoma City, Oklahoma

CHRISTOPHER J. LESSARD, PhD
Assistant Member, Arthritis and Clinical Immunology Research Program, Oklahoma Medical Research Foundation; Department of Pathology, University of Oklahoma Health Sciences Center, Oklahoma City, Oklahoma

RUBEN D. MANTILLA, MD
Center for Autoimmune Diseases Research (CREA), School of Medicine and Health Sciences, Universidad del Rosario, Bogotá, Colombia

XAVIER MARIETTE, MD, PhD
INSERM U1184, Center for Immunology of Viral Infections and Autoimmune Diseases, Université Paris-Sud; Department of Rheumatology, AP-HP, Hôpitaux Universitaires Paris-Sud, Le Kremlin-Bicêtre, France

GAETANE NOCTURNE, MD, PhD
INSERM U1184, Center for Immunology of Viral Infections and Autoimmune Diseases, Université Paris-Sud; Department of Rheumatology, AP-HP, Hôpitaux Universitaires Paris-Sud, Le Kremlin-Bicêtre, France

ANN PARKE, MD, FACR
Professor of Medicine; Division of Rheumatology, St. Francis Hospital and Medical Center, University of Connecticut, Hartford, Connecticut

TOVE RAGNA REKSTEN, PhD
Affiliate, Arthritis and Clinical Immunology Research Program, Oklahoma Medical Research Foundation, Oklahoma City, Oklahoma; Broegelmann Research Laboratory, Department of Clinical Science, University of Bergen, Bergen, Norway

ADRIANA ROJAS-VILLARRAGA, MD
Center for Autoimmune Diseases Research (CREA), School of Medicine and Health Sciences, Universidad del Rosario, Bogotá, Colombia

JUAN CAMILO SARMIENTO-MONROY, MD
Center for Autoimmune Diseases Research (CREA), School of Medicine and Health Sciences, Universidad del Rosario, Bogotá, Colombia

R. HAL SCOFIELD, MD, FACR
Professor, Department of Medicine, College of Medicine, University of Oklahoma Health Sciences Center; Member, Arthritis and Clinical Immunology Program, Oklahoma Medical Research Foundation; Staff Physician, Medical Service, Oklahoma City Department of Veterans Affairs Medical Center, Oklahoma City, Oklahoma

RAPHAÈLE SEROR, MD, PhD
INSERM U1184, Center for Immunology of Viral Infections and Autoimmune Diseases, Université Paris-Sud; Department of Rheumatology, AP-HP, Hôpitaux Universitaires Paris-Sud, Le Kremlin-Bicêtre, France

KATHY L. SIVILS, PhD
Member, Arthritis and Clinical Immunology Research Program, Oklahoma Medical Research Foundation; Department of Pathology, University of Oklahoma Health Sciences Center, Oklahoma City, Oklahoma

FRED K.L. SPIJKERVET, DMD, PhD
Professor and Chairman, Department of Oral and Maxillofacial Surgery, University of Groningen, University Medical Center Groningen, Groningen, The Netherlands

ARJAN VISSINK, DMD, MD, PhD
Professor, Department of Oral and Maxillofacial Surgery, University of Groningen, University Medical Center Groningen, Groningen, The Netherlands

FREDERICK B. VIVINO, MD, MS, FACR
Professor of Clinical Medicine; Chief, Division of Rheumatology, Penn Presbyterian Medical Center, Director, Penn Sjögren's Center, University of Pennsylvania, Philadelphia, Pennsylvania

DAVID T.W. WONG, DMD, DMSc
Professor and Associate Dean of Research, Center for Oral/Head and Neck Oncology Research, School of Dentistry, UCLA, Los Angeles, California

Contents

The management of patients suffering from primary Sjögren syndrome (pSS) has long been mainly symptomatic and demonstration of effectiveness of systemic drugs was lacking. However, progress made in the understanding of pSS pathogenesis has allowed moving into a more targeted approach to therapeutic intervention. Given the key role of chronic B-cell activation, B-cell target therapies were the first candidates. New pathways are currently being investigated, including costimulation and ectopic germinal center. In this review, we summarize the current evidence regarding B-cell targeted and anti-TNF therapies and provide an overview of promising drugs in the pipeline.

We compiled information on antibodies in Sjögren syndrome (SS), focusing more on clinical manifestations associated with anti-Ro/SSA and anti-La/SSB antibodies and studies regarding novel antibodies. We reviewed previous as well as most recent studies with the subject heading Sjogren in combination with antibodies and congenital heart block (CHB). Almost half of asymptomatic mothers giving birth to children with CHB ultimately develop Sjögren. We discussed studies concerning the presence of antibodies predating clinical manifestations of disease. Studies in the future are required to ascertain the pathogenic mechanisms associated with these antibodies and the specific clinical manifestation related to new autoantibodies.

The genes associated with Sjögren syndrome (SS) can be assigned to the NF-kB pathway, the IFN signaling pathway, lymphocyte signaling, and antigen presentation. The frequencies of risk variants show they are common with modest genetic effects. The strongest genetic association outside the human leukocyte antigen region is in IRF5, a gene relevant in the IFN signaling pathway and for B cell differentiation. Although no association has been found with the NF-kB gene itself, associations in TNFAIP3 and TNIP1 (both genome-wide significant), VCAM1 and IRAK1BP (both suggestive), point to genetic explanations for dysregulation of the NF-kB pathway in SS.

Stergios Katsiougiannis and David T.W. Wong

One of the main characteristics of primary Sjögren's syndrome (pSS) is chronic dysfunction and destruction of the salivary and lacrimal glands; their secretory biofluids should reflect the glandular biological status. Saliva is a heterogeneous biofluid comprised of biomolecules and omics constituents that are altered in response to various diseases. Scientific effort has evaluated saliva proteome to diagnose, monitor, and prognosticate pSS. This article reviews the recent advances in salivary proteomics in the context of pSS, highlighting the most significant and promising findings. Determining saliva as a credible means of early disease detection could lead to translational advantages and significant clinical opportunities for pSS.

Juan-Manuel Anaya, Adriana Rojas-Villarraga, Ruben D. Mantilla, Mauricio Arcos-Burgos, and Juan Camilo Sarmiento-Monroy

Polyautoimmunity is defined as the presence of more than one well-defined autoimmune disease (AD) in a single patient. Polyautoimmunity is a frequent condition in Sjögren syndrome (SS) and follows a grouping pattern. The most frequent ADs observed in SS are autoimmune thyroid disease, rheumatoid arthritis, and systemic lupus erythematosus. Main factors associated with polyautoimmunity in SS are tobacco smoking and some genetic variants. The study of polyautoimmunity provides important clues for elucidating the common mechanisms of autoimmne diseases (ie, the autoimmune tautology).

Joana Campos, Maarten R. Hillen, and Francesca Barone

Primary Sjögren's syndrome (pSS) can be considered a systemic autoimmune disease with a strong organ bias. The involvement of the exocrine glands is prevalent and drives the pathognomonic manifestations of dryness that define the sicca syndrome. The salivary glands also represent the hub of pSS pathology. Elements belonging to both innate and acquired immune responses have been described at this site that contribute to disease establishment and progression. The interaction between those elements and their relative contributions to the clinical manifestations and lymphoma progression largely remain to be addressed.

Fred K.L. Spijkervet, Erlin Haacke, Frans G.M. Kroese, Hendrika Bootsma, and Arjan Vissink

Salivary gland biopsy is a technique broadly applied for the diagnosis of Sjögren syndrome (SS), lymphoma in SS, and connective tissue disorders (sarcoidosis, amyloidosis). In SS characteristic histology findings are found, including lymphocytic infiltration surrounding the excretory ducts in combination with destruction of acinar tissue. In this article the main techniques are described for taking labial and parotid salivary gland biopsies with respect to their advantages, postoperative complications, and usefulness for diagnostic procedures, monitoring disease progression, and evaluation of treatment.

Major salivary gland (SG) ultrasonography (US) represents a noninvasive, nonirradiating imaging modality for evaluation of the major SGs in the diagnosis and follow-up of primary and secondary Sjögren syndrome. Structural changes can be visualized as hyperechogenic and hypoechogenic areas, inhomogeneity, and altered echogenicity in general. The reliability of SG-US is poorly investigated, and the definition of US abnormalities varies in previously published studies. Recent studies have shown correlations between SG-US findings and focus score in the minor SGs; however further studies are needed to validate a US criterion in updated classification/diagnostic criteria.

Sjögren syndrome (SS) comprises glandular and extraglandular manifestations. Double-blind prospective trials of traditional disease-modifying antirheumatic drugs and biologics have failed because they have not improved benign symptoms, the major cause of lowered quality of life. Rituximab has proven effective in SS patients with associated mixed cryoglobulinemia, parotid gland swelling, lymphocytic interstitial pneumonitis, thrombocytopenia, and other manifestations. There were few of these SS patients in the trials required for FDA approval. Most patients had benign symptoms and did not show benefit, leading to failure of the study. This article examines the reasons for these failures and proposes future directions.

Sjögren's disease is associated with a high burden of illness, diminished quality of life, and increased health care costs. The Sjögren's Syndrome Foundation developed the first US clinical practice guidelines for management of the oral, ocular, and rheumatologic or systemic manifestations. Guideline recommendations were reviewed by a consensus expert panel using a modified Delphi process. This initiative should improve the quality and consistency of care for Sjögren's disease in the United States, guide insurance reimbursement, and define areas for future study. Guidelines will be periodically reviewed and revised as new information becomes available.

RHEUMATIC DISEASE CLINICS OF NORTH AMERICA

ISSUE OF RELATED INTEREST

Clinics in Chest Medicine, June 2015 (Vol. 36, No. 2)
Chest Imaging
David A. Lynch and Jonathan H. Chung, *Editors*

THE CLINICS ARE AVAILABLE ONLINE!
Access your subscription at:
www.theclinics.com

Foreword

Sjogren's Disease

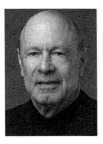

Michael H. Weisman, MD
Consulting Editor

Hal Scofield has done a remarkable job in assembling a timely, up-to-date, and thoughtful review of Sjogren syndrome (SS). It does appear that the science is catching up to the phenomenology that has always characterized this disease. Great strides have been made, and Hal has captured their impact.

Nocturne and colleagues review the data from biologic trials in SS; B-cell targeting has not matched the hopes for its success. However, progress in understanding SS pathogenesis has identified new targets, and trials are underway. Fayyaz and colleagues review the role of autoantibodies attributed to the pathogenesis of SS and attempt to define their exact mechanism of action. Reksten and coworkers discuss the genes associated with SS and the possible role that genetic dysregulation of the NF-kB pathway plays in the pathogenesis of the disease. Katsiougiannis and Wong focus on saliva proteomics in an attempt to validate salivary biomarkers for diagnosis, classification, and prognosis. Anaya and colleagues discuss polyautoimmunity in SS from the standpoint of potential environmental triggers, and Campos and colleagues examine pathologic studies as a key factor in understanding disease establishment and progression. Spijkervet and associates make a strong case for using carefully done parotid gland biopsies as a substitute for the use of minor salivary gland biopsies, and Jonsson and Baldini discuss the emerging role of salivary gland ultrasonography in the diagnosis and management of SS. Bob Fox, with a lifetime of experience in diagnosing and managing patients with SS, provides his insights into why trials have failed by not focusing on what matters most to the patient. Finally,

Rheum Dis Clin N Am 42 (2016) xi–xii
http://dx.doi.org/10.1016/j.rdc.2016.06.002
0889-857X/16/$ – see front matter © 2016 Published by Elsevier Inc.

rheumatic.theclinics.com

Vivino and colleagues review the state-of-the-art of comprehensive management of patients with SS.

Michael H. Weisman, MD
Division of Rheumatology
Cedars-Sinai Medical Center
David Geffen School of Medicine at UCLA
8700 Beverly Boulevard
Los Angeles, CA 90024, USA

E-mail address:
Michael.Weisman@cshs.org

Preface

Sjögren Syndrome in the Twenty-First Century

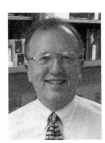

R. Hal Scofield, MD
Editor

Sjögren syndrome is a chronic, systemic autoimmune disease that is common and has important life-altering and severe effects on those with the disease. Despite these facts, the disease has received relatively less attention in terms of research (both laboratory-based and clinical) and in the clinic than related illnesses, such as systemic lupus erythematosus or rheumatoid arthritis. Among the lay public, just about everyone knows someone with lupus it seems, but not so for Sjögren syndrome. As of 23 January 2016, a search of the OVID Medline search engine shows 47,492 articles coded with the MESH Subject Heading "systemic lupus erythematosus" and 86,158 with the MESH Subject Heading "rheumatoid arthritis", but only 10,809 articles coded with the MESH Subject Heading "Sjögren's syndrome". But, perhaps, as evidenced in this issue of *Rheumatic Disease Clinics of North America*, Sjögren syndrome is making up some ground in the early twenty-first century.

As documented by Xavier Mariett and his colleagues, one way in which research in Sjögren is progressing is the study of biologic agents. Furthermore, as noted in this article, there are many ongoing studies with agents tested in other diseases as well as agents that will first be studied in Sjögren syndrome. However, several important trials have either failed or not met their primary endpoint. The provocative article by Robert Fox outlines why it might be that clinical trials in Sjögren syndrome are fraught with difficulty.

There are some clear advantages to the study of Sjögren syndrome. The most obvious of these is the ability of investigators to directly study the affected organs, which lend themselves to biopsy easily. In fact, as emphasized by Barone and colleagues in this issue, the salivary glands are not only the main site of damage in the disease but also the central hub of the pathologic processes. On the other hand, study of the disease has disadvantages. These include difficulty in clinical diagnosis and research classification. The use of both ultrasound and parotid gland biopsy is reviewed in this issue. Neither are part of present research classification criteria, and

Rheum Dis Clin N Am 42 (2016) xiii–xiv
http://dx.doi.org/10.1016/j.rdc.2016.06.001
0889-857X/16/$ – see front matter © 2016 Published by Elsevier Inc.

rheumatic.theclinics.com

neither are ready to be performed widely. Additional research in these areas, however, may lead to important clinical and research use of these techniques. Laboratory-based research to understand the pathologic and etiologic features of the disease is being pursued vigorously as demonstrated in articles reviewing advances in genetics, autoantibodies, and proteomics. Finally, clinical guidelines have recently been issued for treatment of dental and oral disease as well as certain aspects of the systemic illness that occur among those with Sjögren syndrome. Vivino and colleagues have summarized all three of these initial treatment guidelines.

Not included in this issue is a discussion of new classification criteria that are being developed in an alliance of the ACR and EULAR. These new criteria should be published in 2016 and will hopefully provide a unified set of criteria that can be applied to research (including clinical trials) in the disease. I am confident that this issue concentrating on Sjögren syndrome relates the excitement in the field as research and clinical care advance rapidly.

R. Hal Scofield, MD
Department of Medicine
College of Medicine
University of Oklahoma Health Sciences Center
Arthritis and Clinical Immunology Program
Oklahoma Medical Research Foundation
Medical Service
Oklahoma City Department of
Veterans Affairs Medical Center
825 NE 13th Street
Oklahoma City, OK 73104, USA

E-mail address:
hal-scofield@omrf.ouhsc.edu

Use of Biologics in Sjögren's Syndrome

Gaetane Nocturne, MD, PhD[a,b], Divi Cornec, MD, PhD[c,d], Raphaèle Seror, MD, PhD[a,b], Xavier Mariette, MD, PhD[a,b],*

KEYWORDS

- Primary Sjögren's syndrome • Biological treatment • B cell • Clinical trials
- Outcome measure

KEY POINTS

- Consensual indexes have been developed in recent years allowing assessment of disease activity and symptoms in patients with primary Sjögren syndrome (pSS) and thus setting-up of clinical trials.
- Given the key role of B cells in pSS pathogenesis, there was a great deal of hope for B-cell target therapies. But despite promising results from open trials and retrospective studies, rituximab failed to demonstrate efficacy in pSS in 2 randomized controlled studies.
- New pathways are currently being investigated, including specific pathways of B cells, germinal center formation, and costimulation of T cells and interleukin-6.

INTRODUCTION

The management of patients with primary Sjögren syndrome (pSS) has long suffered from the lack of effective treatments. Progress made in the understanding of pSS pathogenesis together with the development of targeted therapies in the rheumatologic field will probably allow moving into the era of biologics in pSS in the near future. B-cell targeted therapies have been the most promising avenue during the past decade. More recently, new targets have been identified and several trials are just about to begin in patients with pSS. A more accurate definition of therapeutic objectives and use of validated outcome measures will help to better identify efficient drugs.

Disclosure Statement: R. Seror received honoraria (less than $10,000) from BMS, GSK, Medlmmune, and Roche; X. Mariette received honoraria (less than $10,000) from BMS, GSK, Medlmmune, and UCB.

[a] INSERM U1184, Center for Immunology of Viral Infections and Autoimmune Diseases, Université Paris-Sud, rue Gabriel Peri, 94270 Le Kremlin-Bicêtre, France; [b] Department of Rheumatology, AP-HP, Hôpitaux Universitaires Paris-Sud, rue du générale Leclerc, 94270 Le Kremlin-Bicêtre, France; [c] Department of Rheumatology, CHRU Brest, rue Boulevard Tanguy Prigent, 29609 Brest, France; [d] EA 2216, INSERM ESPRI, ERI29, Université de Brest, LabEx IGO, 5 Foch - CHU Morvan - BP 824, 29609 Brest, France
* Corresponding author. INSERM U1184, Center for Immunology of Viral Infections and Autoimmune Diseases, Université Paris-Sud, Le Kremlin-Bicêtre, France.
E-mail address: xavier.mariette@aphp.fr

The aim of this article was to summarize efficacy data of biologics used in pSS and to give an overview of the promising drugs in the pipeline.

WHAT ARE THE THERAPEUTIC OBJECTIVES IN PRIMARY SJÖGREN SYNDROME?

Until now, the treatment of pSS mostly relies on symptomatic agents to relieve the main symptoms (tears and saliva substitutes, saliva-stimulating agents such as pilocarpine or cevimeline, and analgesics) and steroids with immunosuppressants in case of severe systemic involvement, but the evidence-based medicine demonstrating the efficacy of these drugs is scarce.[1]

Primary endpoints in the first trials assessing biologics in pSS (tumor necrosis factor [TNF] blockers, rituximab) mainly relied on symptoms, such as the visual analog scale (VAS) for dryness, fatigue, and pain. Even if these manifestations are the most frequent and are responsible for patients' discomfort, they might not represent the only manifestations we want to improve with biologics, and improving systemic manifestations might be a valuable target.

For that purpose, new indexes have been developed to objectively assess systemic and symptomatic manifestations in patients with pSS. The European League Against Rheumatism (EULAR) Sjögren's syndrome disease activity index (ESSDAI) is a systemic disease activity index that was generated in 2009 by consensus of a large group of worldwide experts from European and North American countries.[2] The ESSDAI includes 12 domains (ie, organ systems: cutaneous, respiratory, renal, articular, muscular, peripheral nervous system, central nervous system, hematological, glandular, constitutional, lymphadenopathy, biological). Moderate activity has been defined as an ESSDAI greater than or equal to 5.

Likewise, the EULAR Sjögren's syndrome patient-reported index (ESSPRI) was developed in 2011 in a multicenter international cohort of 230 patients.[3] The selection of domains was based on previous data that included patient interviews,[3,4] and included dryness, pain, and fatigue. The ESSPRI uses 0 to 10 numerical scales, 1 for each domain. The final score is the mean score of the 3 domains.

B-cell Target Therapies

B cell as a central actor of primary Sjögren syndrome pathogeny

Increasing evidence that B cells play a leading role in the disease[5] justified targeting this immune subset in treatment of pSS. In patients with pSS, hypergammaglobulinemia and presence of autoantibodies (rheumatoid factor [RF], anti-SSA/Ro, and anti-SSB/La) support the primary role of B cells. Moreover, B-cell biomarkers have been shown to be increased in patients with pSS.[6] Last, pSS is the autoimmune disease with the higher risk of B-cell non-Hodgkin lymphoma, which represents the ultimate stage of chronic B-cell activation.[7] B-cell activating factor of the TNF family (BAFF) plays a key role in the overstimulation of B cells in pSS. BAFF promotes B-cell maturation, proliferation, and survival, and excess BAFF levels are likely to mediate autoreactive B-cell accumulation.[8] In the past few years, several studies have focused on the role of BAFF in pSS, increased both in the serum and in salivary glands with a correlation between serum BAFF levels with levels of RF and presence of anti-SSA/Ro in patients with pSS.[9] Altogether, these results supported the use of B-cell target therapies in patients with pSS.

Rituximab

Registries and open-labeled studies Rituximab is a chimeric monoclonal antibody targeting CD20, a B-cell–specific membrane protein, that acts through a depletion of mature B cells during 4 to 12 months. Several open-labeled studies including 15 to

30 patients have been conducted to evaluate the efficacy of rituximab in patients with pSS.[10–13] Some of these studies reported an improvement of main pSS symptoms (fatigue, dryness, and pain), as well as quality of life[14] during 6 months following 2 infusions. Longer follow-up suggested that this clinical efficacy was transient.[15] A recent study reported the effects of a much longer and intense exposure to rituximab (5 courses over 2.5 years), and suggested that repeated courses could have a prolonged efficacy.[16]

Other studies reported that rituximab induced a clinically significant improvement in the vast majority of patients with low-grade lymphoma[11] or systemic inflammatory manifestations.[17] The analysis of the French nationwide "AutoImmunité et Rituximab" (AIR) registry reported that rituximab treatment improved systemic manifestations of the disease in 69% of the patients and allowed a decrease of steroid use,[18] especially in case of peripheral nerve involvement associated with cryoglobulinemia or vasculitis.[19] Of note, many of these patients had a severe presentation, and could probably not have been included in a placebo-controlled trial due to the risk of organ damage or even mortality. Thus, these data support the efficacy of rituximab at least in some systemic inflammatory manifestations of pSS-like parotid swelling or cryoglobulinemia-associated vasculitis.

Randomized controlled studies To confirm these findings, 4 randomized controlled studies have been conducted (**Table 1**). The first published trial, performed in the United Kingdom, included only 17 patients and suggested that, among the various symptoms, fatigue was the most likely to be improved by rituximab, even if the primary endpoint was not met.[20] The second study, performed in The Netherlands, included 30 patients (10 assigned to placebo and 20 to rituximab) and reported that stimulated and nonstimulated salivary flow rate was improved 6 months after 2 infusions of 1000 mg[21] in the rituximab arm but not in placebo-treated patients. Two larger multicenter trials were then conducted, the TEARS trial in France[22] and the TRACTISS trial in United Kingsom.[23] The TEARS study included 120 patients with either recent active disease (less than 10 years from disease onset) and biological markers of B-cell hyperactivity, or systemic involvement. Patients received either 2 infusions of 1 g rituximab or a placebo. The primary endpoint (at least 30 mm improvement of at least 2 among 4 VASs assessing global activity by the patient, dryness, fatigue, and pain) was not met at the study completion (week 24), but only at an earlier time point (week 6). However, several other secondary outcome measures were improved, notably salivary flow and salivary gland ultrasonographic abnormalities,[24] raising the possibility that the predefined primary endpoint was not able to measure a positive effect of the treatment. The TRACTISS trial included 133 patients with pSS: 66 were assigned to receive placebo and 67 to rituximab (1000 mg) at weeks 0, 2, 24, and 26. Primary endpoint was the proportion of patients achieving 30% reduction in either fatigue or oral dryness at 48 weeks, measured by VAS. Preliminary results were presented at the 2015 American College of Rheumatology (ACR) meeting in San Francisco: this trial failed to demonstrate any efficacy of rituximab on its primary endpoint: dryness or fatigue VAS, but showed a modest effect of rituximab on salivary flow.[25]

Epratuzumab

Epratuzumab is a humanized immunoglobulin (Ig)G_1-kappa monoclonal antibody targeting CD22, a coreceptor of the B-cell receptor (BCR). Conversely to rituximab, epratuzumab might not act via B-cell depletion. Binding of this molecule to CD22 is likely to enhance CD22 inhibitory functions on BCR and to modulate B-cell activation.[26] Epratuzumab had shown promising results in phase II in patients with moderate/severe

Table 1
Randomized controlled studies of biologicals in primary Sjögren syndrome

Reference	Treatment	N	Primary Endpoint	Significant Difference for Primary Endpoint
Sankar et al,[32] 2004	Etanercept	14	≥20% improvement from baseline for 2 of 3 domains: subjective or objective measures of dry mouth and dry eyes, and IgG level or ESR	No
Mariette et al,[31] 2004 TRIPPS	Infliximab	103	At week 10 ≥30% improvement in 2 of 3 VASs measuring joint pain, fatigue, and the most disturbing dryness.	No and no differences for secondary outcomes
Dass et al,[20] 2008	Rituximab	17	At week 24 20% reduction in VAS fatigue score	No (/placebo) Yes (/baseline)
Meijer et al,[21] 2010	Rituximab	30	At weeks 5, 12, 24, and 48 Improvement in the stimulated whole saliva flow rate	Yes, significant improvement at weeks 5 and 12
Norheim et al,[33] 2012	Anakinra	26	Change in Fatigue VAS at week 4	No
Devauchelle-Pensec et al,[22] 2014 TEARS	Rituximab	122	At week 24 30-mm improvement in 2 of 4 VASs	No, but modest effects on secondary endpoints
Bowman et al,[25] ACR 2015 TRACTISS	Rituximab	110	At 48 wk 30% improvement in VAS fatigue or oral dryness score	No, but modest effect on salivary flow
St Clair et al,[47] 2015	Baminercept, lymphotoxin-beta receptor fusion protein	72	At 24 wk Change in stimulated whole salivary flow	No, but modest effect on ESSDAI

Abbreviations: ACR, American College of Rheumatology; ESR, erythrocyte sedimentation rate; ESS-DAI, European League Against Rheumatism Sjögren's syndrome disease activity index; Ig, immuno-globulin; VAS, visual analog scale.

active lupus.[27] However, results from a phase II randomized controlled trial presented at the 2015 ACR meeting in San Francisco failed to demonstrate any efficacy of epratuzumab in lupus.[28] In pSS, one open-label study including 16 patients who received 4 monthly infusions with epratuzumab reported significant responses in half of the patients.[29] Efficacy was assessed by a composite endpoint involving the Schirmer test, unstimulated whole salivary flow, fatigue, erythrocyte sedimentation rate, and IgG. However, this study was published in 2006, and a randomized trial is mandatory to confirm epratuzumab as a new therapeutic option in pSS.

B-cell activating factor of the tumor necrosis factor family inhibition
Belimumab is a monoclonal antibody targeting BAFF, which has demonstrated its efficacy in the treatment of systemic lupus erythematosus (SLE). The Efficacy and Safety of Belimumab in Subjects With Primary Sjögren's Syndrome (BELISS) study is an open-labeled trial that evaluated efficacy of belimumab in 30 patients with pSS with anti-SSA/Ro and either current systemic complications or salivary gland enlargement, or early disease (<5 years), or biomarkers of B-cell activation.[30] Belimumab was administered at the dosage of 10 mg/kg, at weeks 0, 2, and 4 and then every 4 weeks to week 24. The primary endpoint, assessed at week 28, was improvement in 2 of 5 items: reduction of 30% or more in dryness score on a VAS, 30% or more in fatigue VAS score, 30% or more in VAS pain score, 30% or more in systemic activity VAS assessed by the physician, and/or greater than 25% improvement in any B-cell activation biomarker values. The primary endpoint was achieved by 60% of the patients. Improvement of both patients' symptoms (measured by ESSPRI) and systemic complications (measured by ESSDAI) was observed. Salivary flow and Schirmer test did not change. These results are encouraging, but need to be confirmed in a randomized controlled trial.

TUMOR NECROSIS FACTOR BLOCKERS

Inhibition of TNF has failed to demonstrate efficacy in patients with pSS in 2 randomized controlled studies. In the first one, the Trial of Remicade in Primary Sjögren's Syndrome (TRIPSS) study, 103 patients received infliximab (5 mg/kg) or placebo at weeks 0, 2, and 6 and were followed for 22 weeks.[31] Efficacy, defined as an improvement in 2 of 3 VAS that evaluated pain, fatigue, and dryness, was not achieved. Etanercept was assessed in a 12-week randomized, double-blind, placebo-controlled trial including 28 patients.[32] Again, the primary objective was improvement of VAS for pain, fatigue, and dryness, and etanercept did not lead to a significant improvement of VAS compared with placebo. Blocking of another proinflammatory cytokine, interleukin (IL)-1, has been tested in pSS with the assessment of anakinra, the recombinant IL-1ra, but again, this treatment failed to demonstrate efficacy in patients with pSS.[33]

NEW TARGETS AND FUTURE HOPES
Novel Strategies to Target B Cells

Progress made in the understanding of the pathogeny have allowed the development of new targeted therapies as reported in the **Table 2**. As discussed later in this article, rituximab and belimumab are likely to be powerful therapeutic tools. A better definition of patients who could benefit from these treatments is mandatory. Combination of these 2 drugs could be another therapeutic strategy. Two open-labeled trials assessing this combination in patients with lupus nephritis are currently recruiting (NCT02260934 and NCT02284984), and a randomized double-blind study has just started in patients with pSS (NCT02610543). In addition, a phase II study assessing an anti-BAFF receptor is ongoing in patients with pSS (NCT02149420).

IL-6 plays a key role in terminal B-cell differentiation, B-cell activation, and this cytokine supports the production of IgG. Moreover, IL-6 has been shown to be increased in sera, saliva, and tears of patients with pSS.[34–36] Thus, inhibition of the IL-6 axis

Table 2
Ongoing studies in primary Sjögren syndrome registered on ClincalTrials.gov

Study	Drug	Sponsor	Number of Subjects	Inclusion Criteria	Primary Endpoint	Estimated Completion
NCT02291029	CFZ 533, anti-CD40 monoclonal antibody	Novartis	30	ESSDAI ≥6	ESSDAI change W12	July 2016
NCT02334306	AMG 557/MEDI587, anti-ICOS-L monoclonal antibody	MedImmune/Amgen	42	ESSDAI ≥6 Anti-SSA/SSB and IgG >16 g/L or RF +	ESSDAI change D99	November 2016
NCT01782235 ETAP	Tocilizumab Phase 3	Strasbourg University	110	ESSDAI ≥5 Anti-SSA/SSB	Improvement ESSDAI ≥3	March 2017
NCT02149420	VAY 736, anti-BAFF-R monoclonal antibody	Novartis	30	ESSDAI ≥6 ANA (≥1:160) Anti-SSA/SSB Salivary flow >0	ESSDAI change W12	June 2017
NCT02067910 ASAPIII	Abatacept Phase 3	Gröningen University and BMS	88	ESSDAI ≥5 Disease duration ≤7 Positive parotid biopsy	ESSDAI W24	July 2018
NCT02610543	UCB5857 PI3kinase inhibitor	UCB	58	ESSDAI ≥5 Anti-SSA/SSB Salivary flow >0	ESSDAI change W12	March 2017
NCT02631538	Belimumab/rituximab coadministration	GlaxoSmithKine	70	ESSDAI ≥5 Anti-SSA/SSB Salivary flow >0	Number of participants with SAEs W104	October 2018

Abbreviations: ANA, antinuclear antibodies; BMS, brisол-myers squibb; ESSDAI, European League Against Rheumatism Sjögren's syndrome disease activity index; Ig, immunoglobulin; RF, rheumatoid factor; SAE, severe adverse event; UCB, union chimique belge.

could be interesting in patients with pSS. The ETAP study is a randomized controlled trial assessing safety of tocilizumab, a monoclonal anti-IL6R (NCT01782235). This study is planned to be completed by January 2017.

CD40-CD40 ligand interaction is important for B-cell development, antibody production, germinal center (GC) formation, and optimal T-cell–dependent antibody responses. In patients with pSS, CD40L expression by CD4+ T cells has been shown to be increased compared with controls.[37] A phase II study assessing an anti-CD40 monoclonal antibody is ongoing in pSS (NCT02291029).

Bruton tyrosine kinase (BTK) is involved in the signaling of multiple B-cell molecules, pre-BCR and BCR at the first sight. The key role of BTK in B-cell biology is highlighted by X-linked agammaglobulinemia, which is linked to mutations of BTK. This enzyme has become an attractive therapeutic target in B-cell malignancies.[38,39] BTK is also involved in autoimmune diseases.[40] Mice overexpressing BTK in B cells develop an SLE-like phenotype clinically characterized by kidney, lung, and salivary gland involvement, and biologically characterized by increased GC formation, increased plasma cell number and antinuclear antibody production.[41] Inhibitors of BTK are currently being assessed in rheumatoid arthritis (RA). Assessment in pSS will commence within the near future.

Phosphoinositide 3-kinase (PI3K) plays a key role in the regulation of the immune response. Three classes have been described. PI3K delta belongs to the class IA. In this class, PI3K alpha and beta are ubiquitously expressed, whereas delta is mainly expressed by leukocytes and notably by B cells. It is crucial for mature B-cell development. Interestingly, an inhibitor of this kinase, idelalisib, has shown remarkable efficacy in treating chronic lymphocytic leukemia and non-Hodgkin lymphoma.[42,43] A 12-week proof-of-concept study assessing a new PI3K delta inhibitor in patients with pSS has just started (NCT02610543). Inclusion criteria are defined by ESSDAI of 5 or more, positivity of anti-SSA/SSB, and salivary flow greater than 0. Change of ESSDAI is the primary endpoint.

Germinal Centerlike Structures: A Promising Target

In patients with pSS, GC-like structures are likely to support auto-Ab (anti-SSA/Ro) production.[44] Moreover, GCs have been identified as strong predictors of lymphoma development in pSS.[45] To sum up, these structures support chronic activation of autoimmune B cells. Major advances have been made in the understanding of mechanisms supporting GC-like structure formation and persistence and have helped in identifying new therapeutic targets.[46]

Lymphotoxin

Lymphotoxin has been shown to promote B-cell and T-cell recruitment and high endothelial venule formation within these structures. Baminercept, a lymphotoxin-β receptor IgG1 fusion protein, has been assessed in patients with pSS in a randomized clinical trial. Preliminary results were presented at the 2015 ACR meeting in San Francisco.[47] Primary endpoint was improvement of pilocarpine-stimulated whole salivary flow and was not achieved. However, ESSDAI improved significantly more in the baminercept group than the placebo group. Again, these results highlight the need for better identification of therapeutic objectives in pSS.

CD4 T follicular helper cells

CD4 T follicular helper cells (Tfh) play a crucial role in the persistence of GC-like structures. These cells sustain B-cell activities and notably generation of high-affinity antibodies.[48] Blockade of Tfh signature via inhibition of ICOS (inducible T-cell costimulator)/ICOS-ligand axis or IL-21 signaling, appears promising. Membrane expression of ICOS by Tfh determines their maintenance and controls their anatomic localization in the B-cell follicle. Assessment of an anti-ICOS ligand is ongoing in pSS (NCT02334306). IL-21 is highly expressed by Tfh. IL-21 signaling provides survival and proliferation signals to GC B cells and is a potent inducer of plasma cell differentiation. IL-21 was found to be increased in patients with pSS and is associated with disease activity.[49] Studies assessing an anti-IL-21 antibody were recently completed in lupus (Phase I, NCT01689025) and RA (Phase II, NCT01647451). This new drug also could be relevant in patients with pSS.

T-Cell Costimulation

Abatacept is a fully human soluble fusion protein approved for RA that consists of the extracellular domain of human cytotoxic T-lymphocyte–associated antigen 4 (CTLA-4) linked to the modified Fc portion of human IgG_1. It modulates the CD80/86:CD28 costimulatory signal required for full T-cell activation. To date, 2 open studies have assessed abatacept in pSS. In the first study, 11 patients with pSS received 8 infusions of abatacept. This treatment led to reduction in glandular inflammation and an increase in saliva production.[50] In the ASAP study, 15 patients with pSS received 8 infusions of abatacept.[51] ESSDAI, ESSPRI, RF, and IgG levels decreased significantly but salivary and glandular functions were not modified, underlining the importance of the choice of the primary endpoint for future studies. The ASAPIII study (NCT02067910), a phase III randomized controlled trial, is currently recruiting participants with active disease defined by an ESSDAI of 5 or more. This trial is focused on systemic manifestations of the disease, as the primary endpoint will be ESSDAI improvement.

Type I Interferons

Interferon (IFN) signature is involved in pSS pathogeny. Very recently, it was demonstrated that almost two-thirds of patients with pSS present a high IFN signature. These patients differed from patients with low IFN signature regarding hypergammaglobulinemia, auto-Ab (antinuclear antibody and anti-SSA/Ro), and focus score.[52] These results support the interest of targeting IFN pathways in patients with pSS. However, to date and conversely to what is done in lupus, no anti-IFN biologics have been assessed in pSS. It is known that hydroxychloroquine (HCQ) may inhibit the type I IFN pathway. The randomized controlled JOQUER trial, having included 120 patients with pSS, did not demonstrate any efficacy of HCQ.[52] However, further studies are needed to evaluate impact of anti-IFN drugs on systemic manifestations and longer-term outcomes.

RESEARCH AGENDA

- Progress in the understanding of pSS pathogeny has allowed the development of new target therapies
- B cells, GC-like structures, and T cell costimulation are the most promising perspectives
- Several randomized trials are ongoing for assessing efficacy and safety of drugs targeting these new tools
- Methodological progress in the manner to conduct clinical trials might help to demonstrate treatment efficacy

REFERENCES

1. Ramos-Casals M, Tzioufas AG, Stone JH, et al. Treatment of primary Sjögren syndrome: a systematic review. JAMA 2010;304(4):452–60.

2. Seror R, Ravaud P, Bowman SJ, et al. EULAR Sjögren's syndrome disease activity index: development of a consensus systemic disease activity index for primary Sjögren's syndrome. Ann Rheum Dis 2010;69(6):1103–9.
3. Bowman SJ, Booth DA, Platts RG, et al. Validation of the Sicca symptoms inventory for clinical studies of Sjögren's syndrome. J Rheumatol 2003;30(6):1259–66.
4. Bowman SJ, Booth DA, Platts RG. Measurement of fatigue and discomfort in primary Sjögren's syndrome using a new questionnaire tool. Rheumatology (Oxford) 2004;43(6):758–64.
5. Cornec D, Devauchelle-Pensec V, Tobon GJ, et al. B cells in Sjögren's syndrome: from pathophysiology to diagnosis and treatment. J Autoimmun 2012;39(3): 161–7.
6. Gottenberg JE, Seror R, Miceli-Richard C, et al. Serum levels of beta2-microglobulin and free light chains of immunoglobulins are associated with systemic disease activity in primary Sjögren's syndrome. Data at enrollment in the prospective ASSESS cohort. PLoS One 2013;8(5):e59868.
7. Nocturne G, Mariette X. Sjögren syndrome-associated lymphomas: an update on pathogenesis and management. Br J Haematol 2015;168(3):317–27.
8. Thien M, Phan TG, Gardam S, et al. Excess BAFF rescues self-reactive B cells from peripheral deletion and allows them to enter forbidden follicular and marginal zone niches. Immunity 2004;20(6):785–98.
9. Mariette X, Roux S, Zhang J, et al. The level of BLyS (BAFF) correlates with the titre of autoantibodies in human Sjögren's syndrome. Ann Rheum Dis 2003; 62(2):168–71.
10. Gottenberg JE, Guillevin L, Lambotte O, et al. Tolerance and short term efficacy of rituximab in 43 patients with systemic autoimmune diseases. Ann Rheum Dis 2005;64(6):913–20.
11. Pijpe J, van Imhoff GW, Spijkervet FK, et al. Rituximab treatment in patients with primary Sjögren's syndrome: an open-label phase II study. Arthritis Rheum 2005; 52(9):2740–50.
12. Devauchelle-Pensec V, Pennec Y, Morvan J, et al. Improvement of Sjögren's syndrome after two infusions of rituximab (anti-CD20). Arthritis Rheum 2007;57(2): 310–7.
13. St Clair EW, Levesque MC, Prak ET, et al. Rituximab therapy for primary Sjögren's syndrome: an open-label clinical trial and mechanistic analysis. Arthritis Rheum 2013;65(4):1097–106.
14. Devauchelle-Pensec V, Morvan J, Rat AC, et al. Effects of rituximab therapy on quality of life in patients with primary Sjögren's syndrome. Clin Exp Rheumatol 2011;29(1):6–12.
15. Meijer JM, Pijpe J, Vissink A, et al. Treatment of primary Sjögren syndrome with rituximab: extended follow-up, safety and efficacy of retreatment. Ann Rheum Dis 2009;68(2):284–5.
16. Carubbi F, Cipriani P, Marrelli A, et al. Efficacy and safety of rituximab treatment in early primary Sjögren's syndrome: a prospective, multi-center, follow-up study. Arthritis Res Ther 2013;15(5):R172.
17. Seror R, Sordet C, Guillevin L, et al. Tolerance and efficacy of rituximab and changes in serum B cell biomarkers in patients with systemic complications of primary Sjögren's syndrome. Ann Rheum Dis 2007;66(3):351–7.
18. Gottenberg JE, Cinquetti G, Larroche C, et al. Efficacy of rituximab in systemic manifestations of primary Sjögren's syndrome: results in 78 patients of the Auto-Immune and Rituximab registry. Ann Rheum Dis 2013;72(6):1026–31.

19. Mekinian A, Ravaud P, Hatron PY, et al. Efficacy of rituximab in primary Sjögren's syndrome with peripheral nervous system involvement: results from the AIR registry. Ann Rheum Dis 2012;71(1):84–7.

20. Dass S, Bowman SJ, Vital EM, et al. Reduction of fatigue in Sjögren syndrome with rituximab: results of a randomised, double-blind, placebo-controlled pilot study. Ann Rheum Dis 2008;67(11):1541–4.

21. Meijer JM, Meiners PM, Vissink A, et al. Effectiveness of rituximab treatment in primary Sjögren's syndrome: a randomized, double-blind, placebo-controlled trial. Arthritis Rheum 2010;62(4):960–8.

22. Devauchelle-Pensec V, Mariette X, Jousse-Joulin S, et al. Treatment of primary Sjögren syndrome with rituximab: a randomized trial. Ann Intern Med 2014; 160(4):233–42.

23. Brown S, Navarro Coy N, Pitzalis C, et al. The TRACTISS protocol: a randomised double blind placebo controlled clinical trial of anti-B-cell therapy in patients with primary Sjögren's Syndrome. BMC Musculoskelet Disord 2014;15:21.

24. Jousse-Joulin S, Devauchelle-Pensec V, Cornec D, et al. Brief report: ultrasonographic assessment of salivary gland response to rituximab in primary Sjögren's syndrome. Arthritis Rheumatol 2015;67(6):1623–8.

25. Bowman S, Everett C, Bombardieri M, et al. Preliminary results of a double-blind randomised trial of rituximab anti-B-cell therapy in patients with primary Sjögren's syndrome. Paper presented at: ACR2015. San Francisco, November 6–11, 2015.

26. Sieger N, Fleischer SJ, Mei HE, et al. CD22 ligation inhibits downstream B cell receptor signaling and Ca(2+) flux upon activation. Arthritis Rheum 2013;65(3): 770–9.

27. Wallace DJ, Kalunian K, Petri MA, et al. Efficacy and safety of epratuzumab in patients with moderate/severe active systemic lupus erythematosus: results from EMBLEM, a phase IIb, randomised, double-blind, placebo-controlled, multicentre study. Ann Rheum Dis 2014;73(1):183–90.

28. Clowse MEB, Wallace DJ, Furie R, et al. Efficacy and safety of epratuzumab in patients with moderate-to-severe systemic lupus erythematosus: results from two phase 3 randomized, placebo-controlled trials [abstract]. ACR Meeting. San Francisco: Arthritis Rheumatol. 2015;67 (Suppl 10). 2015.

29. Steinfeld SD, Tant L, Burmester GR, et al. Epratuzumab (humanised anti-CD22 antibody) in primary Sjögren's syndrome: an open-label phase I/II study. Arthritis Res Ther 2006;8(4):R129.

30. Mariette X, Seror R, Quartuccio L, et al. Efficacy and safety of belimumab in primary Sjögren's syndrome: results of the BELISS open-label phase II study. Ann Rheum Dis 2015;74(3):526–31.

31. Mariette X, Ravaud P, Steinfeld S, et al. Inefficacy of infliximab in primary Sjögren's syndrome: results of the randomized, controlled Trial of Remicade in Primary Sjögren's Syndrome (TRIPSS). Arthritis Rheum 2004;50(4):1270–6.

32. Sankar V, Brennan MT, Kok MR, et al. Etanercept in Sjögren's syndrome: a twelve-week randomized, double-blind, placebo-controlled pilot clinical trial. Arthritis Rheum 2004;50(7):2240–5.

33. Norheim KB, Harboe E, Goransson LG, et al. Interleukin-1 inhibition and fatigue in primary Sjögren's syndrome—a double blind, randomised clinical trial. PLoS One 2012;7(1):e30123.

34. Halse A, Tengner P, Wahren-Herlenius M, et al. Increased frequency of cells secreting interleukin-6 and interleukin-10 in peripheral blood of patients with primary Sjögren's syndrome. Scand J Immunol 1999;49(5):533–8.

35. Tishler M, Yaron I, Geyer O, et al. Elevated tear interleukin-6 levels in patients with Sjögren syndrome. Ophthalmology 1998;105(12):2327–9.
36. Tishler M, Yaron I, Shirazi I, et al. Increased salivary interleukin-6 levels in patients with primary Sjögren's syndrome. Rheumatol Int 1999;18(4):125–7.
37. Belkhir R, Gestermann N, Koutero M, et al. Upregulation of membrane-bound CD40L on CD4+ T cells in women with primary Sjögren's syndrome. Scand J Immunol 2014;79(1):37–42.
38. Wang ML, Rule S, Martin P, et al. Targeting BTK with ibrutinib in relapsed or refractory mantle-cell lymphoma. N Engl J Med 2013;369(6):507–16.
39. Wilson WH, Young RM, Schmitz R, et al. Targeting B cell receptor signaling with ibrutinib in diffuse large B cell lymphoma. Nat Med 2015;21(8):922–6.
40. Ponader S, Burger JA. Bruton's tyrosine kinase: from X-linked agammaglobulinemia toward targeted therapy for B-cell malignancies. J Clin Oncol 2014; 32(17):1830–9.
41. Kil LP, de Bruijn MJ, van Nimwegen M, et al. Btk levels set the threshold for B-cell activation and negative selection of autoreactive B cells in mice. Blood 2012; 119(16):3744–56.
42. Furman RR, Sharman JP, Coutre SE, et al. Idelalisib and rituximab in relapsed chronic lymphocytic leukemia. N Engl J Med 2014;370(11):997–1007.
43. Gopal AK, Kahl BS, de Vos S, et al. PI3Kdelta inhibition by idelalisib in patients with relapsed indolent lymphoma. N Engl J Med 2014;370(11):1008–18.
44. Halse AK, Marthinussen MC, Wahren-Herlenius M, et al. Isotype distribution of anti-Ro/SS-A and anti-La/SS-B antibodies in plasma and saliva of patients with Sjögren's syndrome. Scand J Rheumatol 2000;29(1):13–9.
45. Theander E, Vasaitis L, Baecklund E, et al. Lymphoid organisation in labial salivary gland biopsies is a possible predictor for the development of malignant lymphoma in primary Sjögren's syndrome. Ann Rheum Dis 2011;70(8):1363–8.
46. Pitzalis C, Jones GW, Bombardieri M, et al. Ectopic lymphoid-like structures in infection, cancer and autoimmunity. Nat Rev Immunol 2014;14(7):447–62.
47. St Clair EW, Baer AN, Noaiseh G, et al. the clinical efficacy and safety of baminercept, a lymphotoxin-beta receptor fusion protein, in primary Sjögren's syndrome: results from a randomized, double-blind, placebo-controlled phase II trial. ACR Meeting. San Francisco, November 6–11, 2015.
48. Crotty S. Follicular helper CD4 T cells (TFH). Annu Rev Immunol 2011;29:621–63.
49. Gong YZ, Nititham J, Taylor K, et al. Differentiation of follicular helper T cells by salivary gland epithelial cells in primary Sjögren's syndrome. J Autoimmun 2014;51:57–66.
50. Adler S, Korner M, Forger F, et al. Evaluation of histologic, serologic, and clinical changes in response to abatacept treatment of primary Sjögren's syndrome: a pilot study. Arthritis Care Res (Hoboken) 2013;65(11):1862–8.
51. Meiners PM, Vissink A, Kroese FG, et al. Abatacept treatment reduces disease activity in early primary Sjögren's syndrome (open-label proof of concept ASAP study). Ann Rheum Dis 2014;73(7):1393–6.
52. Hall JC, Baer AN, Shah AA, et al. Molecular subsetting of interferon pathways in Sjögren's syndrome. Arthritis Rheumatol 2015;67(9):2437–46.

Autoantibodies in Sjögren's Syndrome

Anum Fayyaz, MBBS[a,b,c], Biji T. Kurien, PhD[a,b,c], R. Hal Scofield, MD[a,b,c],*

KEYWORDS

- Sjögren's syndrome • Autoantibodies • Congenital heart block

KEY POINTS

- Anti-Ro/SSA and anti-La/SSB are commonly found in the sera of patients with Sjögren syndrome and are associated with systemic disease.
- Transplacental transfer of anti-Ro/La causes neonatal lupus and substantial investigation demonstrates pathogenic mechanisms involving these autoantibodies binding neonatal cardiac myositis with induction of inflammation.
- Anti-Ro/La precedes the onset of clinical illness by decades, but thus far no therapeutic intervention is available to prevent disease in healthy antibody-positive individuals who have a high risk of eventually developing the disease.
- Other antibodies found in patients with Sjögren syndrome, such as rheumatoid factor, anti-mitochondrial antibody, and anti-centromere antibody, are associated with particular clinical manifestations.
- Autoantibodies binding the muscarinic 3 receptor affect salivary function and thus are involved in the pathogenicity of the disease.

INTRODUCTION

Sjögren's syndrome is characterized by the presence of a plethora of autoantibodies (**Table 1**). We herein review major recent development in autoantibodies associated with Sjögren syndrome. This includes description of new antibodies found in the sera of patients with the disease as well as clinical associations and new insights into the process by which autoantibodies are produced and are involved in pathogenicity. Animal models of Sjögren syndrome, including autoantibodies, have been reviewed exhaustively in the recent past,[1–3] and are not considered herein.

Disclosures: None.
[a] Arthritis & Clinical Immunology Program, Oklahoma Medical Research Foundation, 825 Northeast, 13th Street, Oklahoma City, OK 73104, USA; [b] Department of Medicine, College of Medicine, 1000 N Lincoln Boulevard, University of Oklahoma Health Sciences Center, Oklahoma City, OK 73104, USA; [c] Medical and Research Services, US Department of Veterans Affairs Hospital, 921 NE 13th Street, Oklahoma City, OK 73104, USA
* Corresponding author. 825 Northeast, 13th Street, Oklahoma City, OK 73104.
E-mail address: Hal-Scofield@omrf.ouhsc.edu

Table 1
Commonly described autoantibodies in Sjögren syndrome

Autoantibodies	Prevalence	Properties	Clinical Association
Anti-Ro/SSA	50%–70%	Disease marker Pathogenic in CHB	Younger age, severe disease Extraglandular, NLS
Anti-La/SSB	25%–40%	Disease marker Pathogenic in CHB	Extraglandular, NLS
RF	36%–74%	Subphenotype marker	Anti-Ro/La, extraglandular
Anti-CCP	3%–10%	Subphenotype marker	Arthritis
AMA	3%–10%	Subphenotype marker	Elevated liver enzymes
ACA	3%–27%	Subphenotype marker	Raynaud phenomenon
Anti-M3R	60%–80%	Potential pathogenic role	Sicca

Anti-Ro/SSA and anti-La/SSB are considered hallmarks of the disease and are associated with systemic disease, but are also present in the sera of patients with SLE. The other listed autoantibodies are more highly associated with other autoimmune diseases but may identify patients with Sjögren's syndrome with certain clinical features. Several other autoantibodies have been more recently described in the disease, but the clinical associations are not yet well delineated (see text under Novel Antibodies).

Abbreviations: ACA, anti-centromere antibody; AMA, anti-mitochondrial antibody; CCP, citrullinated cyclic peptide; CHB, congenital heart block; M3R, muscarinic 3 receptor; NLS, neonatal lupus syndrome; RF, rheumatoid factor.

AUTOANTIBODIES PRECEDE DISEASE

Almost all autoimmune diseases are associated with circulating autoantibodies directed against self-protein. Interestingly many of these disease antibodies are detected years before the clinical manifestations of the disease.[4] Passively acquired autoimmunity substantiated in neonates born to asymptomatic anti-Ro/SSA antibody-positive mothers is one such demonstration.[5] The various manifestations of neonatal lupus syndrome provide a remarkable possibility to explore disease evolution because asymptomatic mothers are brought to medical attention solely on identification of heart block or rash in a neonate.[5–7] Almost half of these asymptomatic mothers ultimately progress to develop some autoimmune ailment with a higher probability toward Sjögren syndrome.[6]

Theander and colleagues[7] recently performed a nested case control study linking data from the Malmo primary Sjögren registry and 3 Swedish health care biobanks. Serum samples were analyzed for antinuclear antibody (ANA), rheumatoid factor (RF), and antibodies against Ro60, Ro52, and La/SSB. Of 117 patients with Sjögren syndrome in the registry who had predisease sera samples available in the biobanks, 81% had autoantibodies before symptom onset.[7,8] Furthermore, many of them had antibodies present in the very earliest available serum sample. Thus, antibodies appeared at least 18 to 20 years before the diagnosis was made.[7,8] The positive predictive value for anti-Ro60 and anti-Ro52 was high for ultimate development of the disease.[7]

Interestingly, these results are consistent with similar studies carried out for systemic lupus erythematosus (SLE) and rheumatoid arthritis (RA).[9,10] In particular, in a study of autoantibodies preceding the diagnosis of SLE in 130 patients diagnosed while in the US Armed Forces, anti-Ro/SSA was among the earliest of antiantibodies to appear with lupus-specific antibodies found closer to the onset of the disease.[9] Congruently, patients with RA have antibodies present years before the diagnosis.[10] Similar data have been generated for other autoimmune diseases, including type

1 diabetes mellitus and primary biliary cirrhosis.[4] Sjögren syndrome, then, falls into a large group of autoimmune diseases in which antibodies precede disease, but the risk of disease in a given antibody-positive individual is not well characterized, except in type 1 diabetes.[4]

ANTI-Ro/SJÖGREN'S SYNDROME A (SSA) AND ANTI-La/SJÖGREN'S SYNDROME B (SSB)

The most common ANAs in patients with Sjögren syndrome are those directed against the autoantigens Ro/SSA and La/SSB.[11–14] The Ro/La particle is a protein-RNA complex formed by the association of the Ro60, and La/SSB proteins with small cytoplasmic RNA (hyRNA).[15] Various methods have been used for the detection of anti-Ro/SSA and anti-La/SSB antibodies. RNA precipitation is considered to be the gold standard method, but other techniques, such as counter-immunoelectrophoresis, immunodiffusion, and enzyme linked immunosorbent assay (ELISA) are more frequently used.[16] It is well to remember that most of the clinical association data for these antibodies in patients with Sjögren syndrome were performed with older assays, such as immunodiffusion, whereas most commercially available assays today are high-throughput, easily automated assays such as ELISA or multiplex bead. These newer assays generally have higher sensitivity and lower specificity; and, thus, associations found with higher specificity, lower sensitivity older assays may not hold true. One study found that the presence of peripheral neuropathy is related to anti-Ro/SSA and anti-La/SSB when determined by precipitation in immunodiffusion but not when determined by ELISA or multiplex bead assay.[17]

Anti-Ro/SSA and anti-La/SSB antibodies are detected in 50% to 70% of patients with primary Sjögren syndrome, depending on the method applied.[18] Anti-Ro/SSA is independent of anti-La/SSB antibody but the contrary is rare,[19] with a recent analysis of the Sjögren's Syndrome International Clinical Alliance cohort concluding that individuals (n = 74) with anti-La/SSB but no anti-Ro/SSA did not have the disease.[20] Data from the Oklahoma Sjögren syndrome cohort support this conclusion (Danda, Kurien, Scofield, manuscript submitted). On the other hand, anti-La/SSB in the presence of anti-Ro/SSA tends to identify patients with Sjögren syndrome. Venables and colleagues[21] found 29 of 35 patients with both anti-Ro/SSA and anti-La/SSB had Sjögren syndrome, whereas among 53 with only anti-Ro/SSA, 23 had Sjögren syndrome, 25 had SLE, and 13 had another disease.

Anti-Ro/SSA and anti-La/SSB antibodies are correlated with younger age at diagnosis, longer disease duration, more severe dysfunction of the exocrine glands, recurrent parotid gland enlargement, and higher intensity of the lymphocytic infiltrates in the minor salivary glands.[22,23] Large studies demonstrate a higher prevalence of extra-glandular manifestations in patients with primary Sjögren syndrome (pSS), including splenomegaly, lymphadenopathy, vasculitis, and Raynaud phenomenon.[24] Sicca-limited disease was found in 292 (29%) of 1010 patients and was associated with an absence of anti-Ro/SSA.[25] This same study found that patients with anti-Ro/La had a lower age at diagnosis, and were statistically more likely to have a host of manifestations. These included parotid enlargement, Raynaud phenomenon, arthritis, vasculitis, renal tubular acidosis, peripheral neuropathy, cytopenias, and RF.[25] A decade long-term study of 100 patients found that only patients with anti-Ro/SSA developed systemic, extraglandular complications.[26]

Patients with Sjögren syndrome are at a marked increased risk for lymphoma, especially mucosal-associated lymphoid tissue (MALT) lymphoma.[27] Despite the increase in incidence, lymphoma is an uncommon event among patients with Sjögren syndrome such that most studies contain a small number of patients. The data concerning the risk of lymphoma in relationship to anti-Ro/SSA and anti-La/SSB are mixed. Studying patients in the north of England with 10-year follow-up, Davidson and colleagues[26] found patients positive for both these antibodies were at high risk for non-Hodgkin lymphoma. Meanwhile, another long-term study with an average of 7 years of follow-up found no difference in serologic testing among the 6 patients who developed lymphoma compared with the 74 who did not.[28] A recent comprehensive review concluded that anti-Ro/La was not a risk factor for lymphoma.[27]

Pulmonary involvement is another complication that may not be associated with the presence of anti-Ro/SSA. A total of 507 patients with Sjögren syndrome underwent chest computed tomography (CT) scan and 50 had bronchiectasis. Only 27% of those with this pulmonary manifestation had anti-Ro/SSA, compared with 54% of those without bronchiectasis.[29] Thus, this serious complication of Sjögren syndrome,[30] unlike most other extraglandular manifestations, is not associated with anti-Ro/SSA. However, this was a study in which all patients underwent a CT scan, and associations may be different when considering patients diagnosed clinically with lung involvement.

The latest biomedical technology continues to be applied to the autoantigenic response to the Ro/SSA and La/SSB proteins. For example, anti-Ro/SSA is strongly associated with increased expression of interferon-regulated genes in peripheral blood mononuclear cells of patients with Sjögren syndrome.[31] Proteomic-based studies to determine V region structures of autoantibodies directed against Ro52 or La/SSB concluded that a set of public clonotypes are used to produce these autoantibodies.[32,33] This same Australian group has conducted proteomic studies of anti-Ro60 that challenge the long-held assumption that these antibodies are produced by long-lived plasma cells. Anti-Ro60 clonotypes in the peripheral blood were determined in 4 patients with Sjögren syndrome over a 7-year period. Immunoglobulin variable gene analysis showed clonotype turnover at approximately 3-month intervals despite long-term high-titer anti-Ro60. Thus, anti-Ro60 was produced by short-lived B cells with rapid turnover.[34] Maier-Moore and colleagues[35] produced recombinant monoclonal antibody from antibody-producing B cells infiltrating the salivary glands of patients with Sjögren syndrome. These studies showed the autoantibody repertoire of the monoclonal antibodies produced from a given subject reflected the antibodies found in the peripheral blood. Thus, this study confirms that the salivary glands are a site for the production of autoantibodies in Sjögren syndrome.[35] The peripheral proteomic study and the salivary gland monoclonal antibody study have not determined the extent to which salivary autoantibody production contributes to circulating anti-Ro60, however.

ANTI-Ro/SSA IN NEONATAL LUPUS

Isolated congenital heart block (CHB) in concert with neonatal lupus dermatitis, hepatitis, and hematologic abnormalities are clinical manifestations of passively acquired autoimmune injury in a neonate; namely, the neonatal lupus syndrome.[5] Third-degree heart block or complete heart block presents a potentially fatal outcome in comparison with other manifestations, which resolve as the maternal antibodies are cleared from the circulatory system of the infant.[36]

Autoimmune CHB occurs in 1% to 2% of anti-Ro/SSA antibody-positive pregnancies, develops in absence of cardiac structural abnormality, and has a recurrence rate of 12% to 20% in subsequent pregnancies.[37,38] CHB is usually diagnosed between weeks 18 and 24 of gestation by fetal echocardiography.[39–43] The association of CHB with maternal autoantibodies to the Ro/SSA autoantigen, which comprises the 2 unrelated proteins, Ro52 and Ro60, is well appreciated.[44,45] A crucial point left unexplained is the low penetrance and recurrence rate of the disease in children of anti-Ro/SSA–positive women, despite persistent maternal antibodies.[37]

The molecular mechanisms underlying CHB pathogenesis are not fully understood. Recently efforts are being invested in delineating a more refined molecular mechanism.[37] CHB is characterized by the presence of immune complex deposits, calcification, and fibrosis at the atrioventricular node in the fetal heart.[44,45] It has to be discerned whether maternal antibodies exert their pathogenic effect by binding their cognate antigen in the heart or whether they cross-react with another molecule on the surface of fetal cardiac cells to directly affect the electrophysiology of the developing heart. Still many reasons have been placed forward to outline a tentative mechanism contributing toward this serious outcome of neonatal lupus.[5]

Ro52 and Ro60 are intracellular proteins. Ro52, which is also known as TRIM21, is a ubiquitin E3 ligase, involved in the regulation of interferon regulatory factor–mediated immune responses, mainly expressed in immune cells.[46–49] Ro60 contributes to RNA quality control.[50] Furthermore, Ro60/TROVE2 promotes cell survival after ultraviolet (UV) irradiation, possibly by assisting in the decay of UV-induced damaged RNA.[51] The mechanism suggested for anti-Ro/SSA antibody binding to its cognate antigen relates to the relocation of Ro60 antigen to the cell surface during apoptosis.[52–54] This observation led to the apoptosis-inflammation hypothesis,[37] which postulates that maternal anti-Ro/SSA antibodies bind to apoptotic cardiac cells during the normal remodeling in the developing heart. This leads to diversion from a noninflammatory to an inflammatory pathway.[37,55] In vitro studies have demonstrated that opsonized apoptotic cardiocytes can eventually activate phagocytic cells to produce proinflammatory and profibrotic cytokines that ultimately result in atrioventricular (AV) node scarring.[55,56] Translocation of the Ro/SSA and La/SSB antigens to the cell surface in the salivary gland during apoptosis also has been invoked as a mechanism of Sjögren syndrome in general, which involves activation of epithelial cells.[57–60]

Anti-Ro52 antibodies induce AV block in several animal models of CHB.[61] These antibodies have been found in the vast majority of mothers giving birth to children with CHB. Boutjdir and colleagues[62] in the late 1990s demonstrated a direct effect of maternal autoantibodies on the heart conduction system. By perfusing rat hearts with isolated fractions of immunoglobulin (Ig)G from the maternal serum, and dissecting atrial and AV nodal areas of rat heart, this study demonstrated bradycardia with AV nodal block. Most recently, the fine specificity of the anti-Ro52 response has been shown to correlate with complete CHB by Salomonsson and colleagues.[63] By study of maternal antibodies directed to a specific epitope within the leucine zipper amino acid sequence 200 to 239 (p200) of the Ro52 protein, this group showed prolongation of fetal AV nodal time and AV block, while antibodies targeting other domains of Ro52 did not lead to such changes. The mechanism delineated by these experiments showed anti-Ro/SSA binding cell surface type E calcium channels with resultant effect on Ca^{2+} oscillations, leading to accumulating levels and overload of intracellular Ca^{2+} levels with subsequent loss of contractility and ultimately apoptosis.[63] But, the role of anti-Ro52 antibodies as the sole drivers in the pathogenesis of CHB has yet to be proven.

CHB recurrence rates are at most 20% in a subsequent pregnancy, indicating that factors beyond maternal antibody profile are involved in CHB. Reed and colleagues[64] demonstrated that β-2 glycoprotein 1 (β2GP1) prevented opsonization of apoptotic cardiomyocytes by maternal anti-Ro60 IgG. This can be considered in relation to the "apoptotic" theory of cardiac neonatal lupus, in which the formation of pathogenic antibody-apoptotic cell immune complexes promotes proinflammatory and profibrotic responses. Briassouli and colleagues[65] demonstrated that transforming growth factor

(TGF)-beta is triggered by immune reactions leading to amplification of TGF inducing a cascade of events that promotes myofibroblast transdifferentiation and scar formation. Finally, genetic association has been demonstrated for CHB.

RHEUMATOID FACTOR

RF is commonly found in the sera of patients with Sjögren syndrome and is associated with serologic positivity for anti-Ro/SSA and anti-La/SSB as well as systemic disease.[66] Recent reports continue to support these associations. In a study of 212 patients with Sjögren syndrome, only anti-Ro/SSA, anti-La/SSB, hypergammaglobulinemia, and RF were associated with systemic disease and use of corticosteroid.[67] Similarly, a large Italian study found RF was one of only a few markers for severe disease.[68] The relationship of RF to systemic disease is found in all racial and ethnic groups studied.[69] One small study found excess pulmonary disease among patients with RF,[70] whereas IgA RF was associated with renal disease in another cohort.[71] The presence of RF was a marker of more severe exocrine gland manifestations (keratoconjunctivitis sicca) among 121 patients with Sjögren syndrome followed for at least 1 year.[72] Thus, RF is a prognostic finding in Sjögren syndrome but may not be useful for clinical diagnosis or research classification purposes because this antibody is found commonly in other diseases.

ANTI-MUSCARINIC RECEPTOR AUTOANTIBODIES

Salivary flow is a result of neural stimulation of the acinar and ductal cells of the glands, specifically in response to muscarinic/cholinergic receptor agonists. The presence of functional autoantibodies against glandular M3 muscarinic acetylcholine receptors (M3R) has been reported in pSS. However, the pathogenic role of these autoantibodies in Sjögren syndrome development remains to be unraveled. Robinson and colleagues[73] in 1998 transferred immunoglobulin from anti-Ro/SSA–positive patients with Sjögren syndrome into mice that lacked native immunoglobulin. This study showed reduction of salivary flow in the mice receiving patient immunoglobulin. Their study demonstrated antibody that affected exocrine gland function and that this affect potentially was mediated by binding muscarinic receptors. Hence, this study supports the concept that antibodies directed against autonomic nervous system receptors play a central role in the clinical manifestation of Sjögren syndrome.

Borda and colleagues have been working over many years to elucidate the pathogenic mechanisms associated with anti-M3R autoantibodies contributing to the clinical manifestation of Sjögren syndrome. These investigators demonstrated that primary patients with Sjögren syndrome produce functional IgG autoantibodies that interact with M3R. IgG from patients has 2 effects on the submandibular gland. The antibodies can act as an inducer of the proinflammatory molecule prostaglandin E_2 (PGE_2), which in turn inhibits Na^+/K^+-ATPase activity.[74] Antibodies may also have a role in the pathogenesis of dry mouth by Na^+/K^+-ATPase inhibition and the net K^+ efflux stimulation of the salivary gland in response to the authentic agonist pilocarpine, decreasing salivary fluid production. The same group demonstrated serum IgG from patients with Sjögren syndrome, interact with the second extracellular loop of human glandular M3R, triggering the production of matrix metalloproteinase-3 (MMP-3) and prostaglandin E_2.[75] Thus, Borda and colleagues propose that PGE2 and MMP-3 are generated by autoantibody activation of COX-2. Hence, an imbalance in the expression and activity of PGE_2 and MMP-3 may lead to severe dysfunction of the salivary glands.[75]

In a recent study involving 24 Sjögren syndrome subjects, Kim and colleagues[76] investigated the pathologic role of autoantibodies associated with downregulation of the major histocompatibility complex I (MHC I) molecule through M3R internalization. The study implicated this action as an important mechanism contributing to the impaired salivation seen in Sjögren syndrome. This study also showed that MHC I did not directly interact with Sjögren syndrome IgG, validating the presence of specific anti-M3R autoantibodies in pSS. The Sjögren syndrome IgG-induced internalization of M3R with MHC I was significantly inhibited by the cholesterol-sequestering drug filipin. The fact that filipin significantly inhibited autoantibody-induced internalization of M3R with MHC I suggests a potential therapeutic for patients with pSS.[76]

Park and colleagues[77] studied the role of functional anti-M3R antibodies in gastrointestinal (GI) dysfunction associated with pSS.[77] Using muscle strip and whole-organ functional assays, this study determined whether anti-M3R antibodies disrupted neurotransmission in tissue throughout the mouse GI tract. The effect of the IgG on GI tissue was dependent on expression of the M3R, demonstrating for the first time a role for autoantibodies specific for this receptor mediate autonomic dysfunction in pSS.

However, there is no consensus regarding the presence or role of anti-M3R in Sjögren syndrome or method of detection. In 2001, Bacman and colleagues[78] used synthetic 25-mer peptide, corresponding to the second extracellular loop of human M3R, as an antigen to demonstrate molecular interaction with autoantibodies from sera of primary and secondary patients with Sjögren syndrome. However, Cavill and colleagues[79] challenged the method of determination in Bacman's study. Waterman and colleagues[80] used functional assays to investigate autoantibody-mediated effects on parasympathetic neurotransmission and smooth muscle contraction in their studies, and suggest that synthetic peptide is a linear structure that does not reproduce the actual in vivo configuration of the epitope. These investigators advocate that simple peptide-based immunoassays cannot replace complex functional assays for detection of anti-M3R antibodies.[79]

ANTI-CENTROMERE ANTIBODY

Anti-centromere antibodies (ACAs) have been increasingly studied in context of Sjögren syndrome. Although ACAs are commonly found among patients with limited cutaneous scleroderma, studies have been carried out relating Sjögren syndrome to ACA. The prevalence of ACA in primary Sjögren syndrome ranges from 3.7% to 27.0% when detected by indirect immunofluorescence, and from 20% to 25% when detected by other methods.[81,82] In a study of 1323 sera from patients with a wide variety of connective tissue disease, the most common clinical manifestation associated with ACA was Raynaud phenomenon.[83] Retrospectively, Renier and colleagues[84] reported a strikingly high prevalence of sicca manifestations (76%) among 67 patients positive for ACA. In 41 patients positive for ACA derived from a population of 2627 subjects in a prospective study, primary Sjögren syndrome was diagnosed in 7 (17%) of this outpatient population.[85] This study, for the first time, established an association between primary Sjögren syndrome and ACA.[85]

The staining of the centromere region of cells in indirect immunofluorescence by autoantibodies in human sera was first described in 1980.[86] Immunoblotting of the nuclear extracts revealed the 3 major polypeptide antigens recognized by ACA, designated CENP-A, CENP-B, and CENP-C.[87] Anti-CENP-B and anti-CENP-C antibodies recognize granzyme B–generated fragments, which suggested a role for granzyme-B–bearing cytotoxic cells in pathogenesis.[88]

The pattern of CENP recognition differs markedly in primary Sjögren syndrome and limited scleroderma. Patients with primary Sjögren syndrome predominantly recognize CENP-C alone, whereas dual recognition of CENP-B and CENP-C is most frequently seen in scleroderma. Pillemer and colleagues,[89] in 2004, studying sera from 45 patients with Sjögren syndrome to determine which centromere protein is recognized and to identify a specific serologic subset, concluded antibodies binding both CENP-B and CENP-C does occur. Pillemer and colleagues[89] hypothesized that patients with pSS with serum antibodies to certain centromere proteins represent a distinct clinical subset of the Sjögren syndrome population. Gelber and colleagues[90] in 2006 studied whether distinct centromere proteins are targeted in pSS and scleroderma. Sera from 45 patients with pSS and 33 with limited scleroderma were studied. Ten of 45 patients with pSS and 18 of 33 with scleroderma had antibodies recognizing CENPs. Seven (70%) of 10 patients positive for CENP with pSS recognized CENP-C alone, compared with 1 (6%) of 18 patients positive for CENP with limited scleroderma. Thus, the pattern of CENP recognition differed between pSS and limited scleroderma.[90]

Kitagawa and colleagues[70] described the clinical features of ACA-positive patients with pSS and suggested including ACA in the classification criteria. In this study, during a 6.5-year period, 64 patients were diagnosed with pSS, and 3 groups were established based on ACA. In the ACA(+) group, there were high positive rates for both abnormal Schirmer test and fluorescein staining of the cornea, similar to those in the Ro/SSA(+) group and Ro/SSA-La/SSB(+) group. Thus, according to this study, ACA is an autoantibody that reflects the degree of impaired salivary and lacrimal gland function. The UK Primary Sjögren Syndrome Registry established by Collins and colleagues[91] had contrasting results to Kitagawa and colleagues.[70] According to this study, if ACA were incorporated in the classification criteria, only 3 of 87 anti-Ro/La–negative patients could have avoided minor salivary gland biopsy. The study concluded the prevalence of ACA was not significant enough to incorporate ACA positivity in the classification criteria for pSS.

Ramos-Casals and colleagues[92] studied ACA among 402 patients with Sjögren syndrome. Using ELISA as the method of detection, 8 (2.0%) had ACA. Raynaud phenomenon (n = 6) and pulmonary involvement (n = 3) were common, whereas anti-Ro/SSA and anti-La/SSB were present in only 1 of the 8 ACA-positive patients. Three of the 8 developed features consistent with limited scleroderma. These 3 had Raynaud phenomenon, high-titer ANA, no anti-Ro/SSA, or anti-La/SSB with development of sclerodactyly.

OTHER AUTOANTIBODIES IN SJÖGREN SYNDROME

Autoantibodies against cyclic citrullinated peptides (anti-CCP) in patients with Sjögren syndrome have been estimated to range between 3% and 10%.[93–95] In Sjögren syndrome, the presence of these autoantibodies has been related to nonerosive arthritis.[96] However, a French study found 10 of 134 patients with pSS not meeting criteria for RA had anti-CCP but found no difference in clinical features.[94] In addition, 9 additional patients with Sjögren syndrome who also fulfilled the American College of Rheumatology RA criteria all had anti-CCP.[94]

Antimitochondrial antibodies (AMA) are reportedly present in 1.7% to 13.0% of patients with Sjögren syndrome, with the rate rising to 3% to 27% depending on the diagnostic method applied.[97] AMAs serve as a serologic marker of primary biliary cirrhosis. The 2 diseases are both characterized by inflammation of epithelium. Selmi and colleagues[97] proposed primary biliary cirrhosis can be considered as Sjögren syndrome of the liver and Sjögren syndrome as primary biliary cirrhosis of the salivary glands. Association of liver involvement in Sjögren syndrome with serum AMA has been reported, but liver enzymes can be elevated without AMA. Also, characteristic symptoms of Sjögren syndrome, such as dry mouth or dry eyes are commonly found in primary biliary cirrhosis, but anti-Ro/SSA is rarely observed. Hence, further studies are mandated to relate AMA to specific clinical features in SS.

A study of atypical antibodies among 402 patients with Sjögren syndrome found 82 (20%) with at least 1 of anti-DNA (n = 21), anti-RNP (n = 10), anti-Sm (n = 6), anti-SCL70 (n = 2), ACA (n = 6), anti-Jo-1 (n = 1), anti-neutrophil cytoplasmic (n = 13), or anti-cardiolipin (n = 36).[92] The only clinical feature different between these patients and those without such antibodies was an increased prevalence of Raynaud phenomenon, which was driven by those patients with ACA. In moderate-term follow-up, 13 of the 82 went on to develop another autoimmune disease, usually characteristic of the "atypical" antibody found in their sera, whereas those without these antibodies did not do so.[92] Our group has reported a patient with Sjögren syndrome with anti-PL12 (associated with anti-synthetase syndrome) in which anti-PL12 was produced by B cells infiltrating the salivary gland.[35]

Patients with Sjögren syndrome have antibodies directed against α-fodrin, the non-erythroid homolog of spectrin.[98] But the specificity and importance of these antibodies has been questioned. Anti-α-fodrin was observed in almost twice as many patients with non–Sjögren syndrome sicca compared with subjects with Sjögren syndrome having anti-Ro60, anti-La, and sicca.[99] Similarly, Nordmark and colleagues[100] observed anti-α-fodrin antibodies in 29% (16/56) of patients with pSS and in 47% (25/53) of patients with SLE (without secondary Sjögren syndrome), but in only 21% (3/14) of SLE with secondary Sjögren syndrome . These investigators suggest that α-fodrin autoantibodies have no discriminating value and are mainly related to non–organ-specific autoimmunity in primary Sjögren syndrome , SLE, and non–Sjögren syndrome sicca.[100] Zandbelt and colleagues[101] found that anti-Ro60 and anti-La/SSB to be more sensitive for Sjögren syndrome diagnosis than α-fodrin antibodies in ELISA, as well as other methods.

Thus, the anti-fodrin is found in patients with Sjögren syndrome but also in individuals with SLE as well as those with non–Sjögren syndrome sicca. We conclude that anti-fodrin is not useful for diagnosis in Sjögren syndrome, as the presence of these antibodies cannot distinguish patients with Sjögren syndrome from those with non–Sjögren syndrome sicca.

NOVEL ANTIBODIES

Recently many studies have been carried out to analyze novel autoantibodies. Nozawa and colleagues[102] analyzed the prevalence of autoantibodies to NA14, which were observed mostly in pSS. Their data, from sera collected in patients with various rheumatic diseases from cohorts in both the United States and Japan, showed a substantial fraction, 36.4% (4/11) of anti-NA14–positive sera, was negative for anti-Ro/SSA and anti-La/SSB antibodies.

Studying sera from 46 patients with SLE but without Sjögren syndrome, 11 patients with SLE with secondary Sjögren syndrome, and 45 patients with pSS, Matsushita and colleagues[103] evaluated anti-proteasome activator (anti-PA28a) antibodies as anti-cytoplasmic antibodies in Sjögren syndrome. Anti-PA28a antibodies were found to be present in 40% of the anti-Ro/SSA–positive patients, and the incidence was higher than those of anti-ribosomal P, anti–smooth muscle, and anti-mitochondrial antibodies. The study concluded further evaluation of clinical significance of anti-PA28a antibody was mandatory.[103]

Shen and colleagues[104] recognized new antibodies, namely, salivary gland protein 1 (SP-1), carbonic anhydrase 6 (CA6), and parotid secretory protein (PSP) associated with Sjögren syndrome–like illness in animal models, patients with established disease, and in patients with idiopathic xerostomia and xerophthalmia. In humans, this work evaluated sera of 13 patients with established disease; 62% had antibodies to Ro/SSA or La/SSB, 54% had antibodies to SP-1, 54% had antibodies to CA6, and 69% had antibodies to SP-1 or CA6. In addition, 45% of those with a positive salivary gland biopsy but no anti-Ro/SSA or anti-La/SSB had antibodies to SP-1, whereas 5% had antibodies to CA6.[104] Further studies are required to develop understanding regarding the clinical importance and associations of these new antibodies. Replication by others of these findings will be important given the small number of patients studied.

Wolska and colleagues,[105] in a very recent study, showed that autoantibodies targeting TRIM38 (along with R052, a member of family of TRIM proteins) were present in approximately 10% of patients with pSS. The presence of these autoantibodies was also associated with overall higher severity of disease.

SUMMARY

The study of autoantibodies in Sjögren syndrome is alive and well. Many studies are being carried out to discern pathologic attributions of disease-associated autoantibodies. A pathogenic role for anti-Ro/SSA and/or anti-La/SSB is known in autoimmune CHB, and work is being carried out to define the mechanism for the pathologic role. Although antibodies preceding disease provide an opportunity to identify and study subjects before disease onset, interventions at this stage have not been developed. New autoantibodies open a window for making additions to the diagnostic approach but no emerging antibody is as yet ready for a role in the clinic.

REFFRENCES

1. Lavoie TN, Lee BH, Nguyen CQ. Current concepts: mouse models of Sjögren's syndrome. J Biomed Biotechnol 2011;2011:549107.
2. Donate A, Voigt A, Nguyen CQ. The value of animal models to study immunopathology of primary human Sjögren's syndrome symptoms. Expert Rev Clin Immunol 2014;10(4):469–81.
3. Delaleu N, Nguyen CQ, Peck AB, et al. Sjögren's syndrome: studying the disease in mice. Arthritis Res Ther 2011;13(3):217.
4. Scofield RH. Autoantibodies as predictors of disease. Lancet 2004;363(9420): 1544–6.
5. Buyon J, Szer I. Passively acquired autoimmunity and the maternal fetal dyad in systemic lupus erythematosus. Springer Semin Immunopathol 1986;9(2–3): 283–304.
6. Rivera TL, Izmirly PM, Birnbaum BK, et al. Disease progression in mothers of children enrolled in the Research Registry for Neonatal Lupus. Ann Rheum Dis 2009;68(6):828–35.
7. Theander E, Jonsson R, Sjostrom B, et al. Prediction of Sjögren's syndrome years before diagnosis and identification of patients with early onset and severe

disease course by autoantibody profiling. Arthritis Rheumatol 2015;67(9): 2427–36.

8. Jonsson R, Theander E, Sjostrom B, et al. Autoantibodies present before symptom onset in primary Sjögren syndrome. JAMA 2013;310(17):1854–5.

9. Arbuckle MR, McClain MT, Rubertone MV, et al. Development of autoantibodies before the clinical onset of systemic lupus erythematosus. N Engl J Med 2003; 349(16):1526–33.

10. Nielen MM, van Schaardenburg D, Reesink HW, et al. Specific autoantibodies precede the symptoms of rheumatoid arthritis: a study of serial measurements in blood donors. Arthritis Rheum 2004;50(2):380–6.

11. Skopouli FN, Dafni U, Ioannidis JP, et al. Clinical evolution, and morbidity and mortality of primary Sjögren's syndrome. Semin Arthritis Rheum 2000;29(5): 296–304.

12. ter Borg EJ, Risselada AP, Kelder JC. Relation of systemic autoantibodies to the number of extraglandular manifestations in primary Sjögren's Syndrome: a retrospective analysis of 65 patients in the Netherlands. Semin Arthritis Rheum 2011; 40(6):547–51.

13. Fauchais AL, Martel C, Gondran G, et al. Immunological profile in primary Sjögren syndrome: clinical significance, prognosis and long-term evolution to other auto-immune disease. Autoimmun Rev 2010;9(9):595–9.

14. Nardi N, Brito-Zeron P, Ramos-Casals M, et al. Circulating auto-antibodies against nuclear and non-nuclear antigens in primary Sjögren's syndrome: prevalence and clinical significance in 335 patients. Clin Rheumatol 2006;25(3): 341–6.

15. Keene JD. Molecular structure of the La and Ro autoantigens and their use in autoimmune diagnostics. J Autoimmun 1989;2(4):329–34.

16. Franceschini F, Cavazzana I. Anti-Ro/SSA and La/SSB antibodies. Autoimmunity 2005;38(1):55–63.

17. Scofield AK, Radfar L, Ice JA, et al. Relation of sensory peripheral neuropathy in Sjögren syndrome to anti-Ro/SSA. J Clin Rheumatol 2012;18(6):290–3.

18. Vitali C, Bootsma H, Bowman SJ, et al. Classification criteria for Sjögren's syndrome: we actually need to definitively resolve the long debate on the issue. Ann Rheum Dis 2013;72(4):476–8.

19. Elkon KB, Gharavi AE, Hughes GR, et al. Autoantibodies in the sicca syndrome (primary Sjögren's syndrome). Ann Rheum Dis 1984;43(2):243–5.

20. Baer AN, McAdams DeMarco M, Shiboski SC, et al. The SSB-positive/SSA-negative antibody profile is not associated with key phenotypic features of Sjögren's syndrome. Ann Rheum Dis 2015;74(8):1557–61.

21. Venables PJ, Shattles W, Pease CT, et al. Anti-La (SS-B): a diagnostic criterion for Sjögren's syndrome? Clin Exp Rheumatol 1989;7(2):181–4.

22. Manoussakis MN, Pange PJ, Moutsopulos HM. The autoantibody profile in Sjögren's syndrome. Ter Arkh 1988;60(4):17–20 [in Russian].

23. Mavragani CP, Tzioufas AG, Moutsopoulos HM. Sjögren's syndrome: autoantibodies to cellular antigens. Clinical and molecular aspects. Int Arch Allergy Immunol 2000;123(1):46–57.

24. Tzioufas AG, Wassmuth R, Dafni UG, et al. Clinical, immunological, and immunogenetic aspects of autoantibody production against Ro/SSA, La/SSB and their linear epitopes in primary Sjögren's syndrome (pSS): a European multi-centre study. Ann Rheum Dis 2002;61(5):398–404.

25. Ramos-Casals M, Solans R, Rosas J, et al. Primary Sjögren syndrome in Spain: clinical and immunologic expression in 1010 patients. Medicine (Baltimore) 2008;87(4):210–9.

26. Davidson BK, Kelly CA, Griffiths ID. Primary Sjögren's syndrome in the North East of England: a long-term follow-up study. Rheumatology (Oxford) 1999; 38(3):245–53.

27. Papageorgiou A, Voulgarelis M, Tzioufas AG. Clinical picture, outcome and predictive factors of lymphoma in Sjögren syndrome. Autoimmun Rev 2015;14(7): 641–9.

28. Gannot G, Lancaster HE, Fox PC. Clinical course of primary Sjögren's syndrome: salivary, oral, and serologic aspects. J Rheumatol 2000;27(8):1905–9.

29. Soto-Cardenas MJ, Perez-De-Lis M, Bove A, et al. Bronchiectasis in primary Sjögren's syndrome: prevalence and clinical significance. Clin Exp Rheumatol 2010;28(5):647–53.

30. Kreider M, Highland K. Pulmonary involvement in Sjögren syndrome. Semin Respir Crit Care Med 2014;35(2):255–64.

31. Emamian ES, Leon JM, Lessard CJ, et al. Peripheral blood gene expression profiling in Sjögren's syndrome. Genes Immun 2009;10(4):285–96.

32. Arentz G, Thurgood LA, Lindop R, et al. Secreted human Ro52 autoantibody proteomes express a restricted set of public clonotypes. J Autoimmun 2012; 39(4):466–70.

33. Thurgood LA, Arentz G, Lindop R, et al. An immunodominant La/SSB autoantibody proteome derives from public clonotypes. Clin Exp Immunol 2013;174(2): 237–44.

34. Lindop R, Arentz G, Bastian I, et al. Long-term Ro60 humoral autoimmunity in primary Sjögren's syndrome is maintained by rapid clonal turnover. Clin Immunol 2013;148(1):27–34.

35. Maier-Moore JS, Koelsch KA, Smith K, et al. Antibody-secreting cell specificity in labial salivary glands reflects the clinical presentation and serology in patients with Sjögren's syndrome. Arthritis Rheumatol 2014;66(12):3445–56.

36. Waltuck J, Buyon JP. Autoantibody-associated congenital heart block: outcome in mothers and children. Ann Intern Med 1994;120(7):544–51.

37. Ambrosi A, Sonesson SE, Wahren-Herlenius M. Molecular mechanisms of congenital heart block. Exp Cell Res 2014;325(1):2–9.

38. Brucato A, Frassi M, Franceschini F, et al. Risk of congenital complete heart block in newborns of mothers with anti-Ro/SSA antibodies detected by counterimmunoelectrophoresis: a prospective study of 100 women. Arthritis Rheum 2001;44(8):1832–5.

39. Buyon JP, Hiebert R, Copel J, et al. Autoimmune-associated congenital heart block: demographics, mortality, morbidity and recurrence rates obtained from a national neonatal lupus registry. J Am Coll Cardiol 1998;31(7):1658–66.

40. Solomon DG, Rupel A, Buyon JP. Birth order, gender and recurrence rate in autoantibody-associated congenital heart block: implications for pathogenesis and family counseling. Lupus 2003;12(8):646–7.

41. Julkunen H, Eronen M. The rate of recurrence of isolated congenital heart block: a population-based study. Arthritis Rheum 2001;44(2):487–8.

42. Llanos C, Izmirly PM, Katholi M, et al. Recurrence rates of cardiac manifestations associated with neonatal lupus and maternal/fetal risk factors. Arthritis Rheum 2009;60(10):3091–7.

43. Ambrosi A, Salomonsson S, Eliasson H, et al. Development of heart block in children of SSA/SSB-autoantibody-positive women is associated with maternal age and displays a season-of-birth pattern. Ann Rheum Dis 2012;71(3):334–40.

44. Litsey SE, Noonan JA, O'Connor WN, et al. Maternal connective tissue disease and congenital heart block. Demonstration of immunoglobulin in cardiac tissue. N Engl J Med 1985;312(2):98–100.

45. Lee LA, Coulter S, Erner S, et al. Cardiac immunoglobulin deposition in congenital heart block associated with maternal anti-Ro autoantibodies. Am J Med 1987;83(4):793–6.

46. Espinosa A, Zhou W, Ek M, et al. The Sjögren's syndrome-associated autoantigen Ro52 is an E3 ligase that regulates proliferation and cell death. J Immunol 2006;176(10):6277–85.

47. Espinosa A, Dardalhon V, Brauner S, et al. Loss of the lupus autoantigen Ro52/Trim21 induces tissue inflammation and systemic autoimmunity by disregulating the IL-23-Th17 pathway. J Exp Med 2009;206(8):1661–71.

48. Yoshimi R, Chang TH, Wang H, et al. Gene disruption study reveals a nonredundant role for TRIM21/Ro52 in NF-kappaB-dependent cytokine expression in fibroblasts. J Immunol 2009;182(12):7527–38.

49. Yang K, Shi HX, Liu XY, et al. TRIM21 is essential to sustain IFN regulatory factor 3 activation during antiviral response. J Immunol 2009;182(6):3782–92.

50. Chen X, Wolin SL. The Ro 60 kDa autoantigen: insights into cellular function and role in autoimmunity. J Mol Med (Berl) 2004;82(4):232–9.

51. Chen X, Smith JD, Shi H, et al. The Ro autoantigen binds misfolded U2 small nuclear RNAs and assists mammalian cell survival after UV irradiation. Curr Biol 2003;13(24):2206–11.

52. Casciola-Rosen LA, Anhalt G, Rosen A. Autoantigens targeted in systemic lupus erythematosus are clustered in two populations of surface structures on apoptotic keratinocytes. J Exp Med 1994;179(4):1317–30.

53. Miranda ME, Tseng CE, Rashbaum W, et al. Accessibility of SSA/Ro and SSB/La antigens to maternal autoantibodies in apoptotic human fetal cardiac myocytes. J Immunol 1998;161(9):5061–9.

54. Reed JH, Neufing PJ, Jackson MW, et al. Different temporal expression of immunodominant Ro60/60 kDa-SSA and La/SSB apotopes. Clin Exp Immunol 2007;148(1):153–60.

55. Clancy RM, Kapur RP, Molad Y, et al. Immunohistologic evidence supports apoptosis, IgG deposition, and novel macrophage/fibroblast crosstalk in the pathologic cascade leading to congenital heart block. Arthritis Rheum 2004;50(1):173–82.

56. Clancy RM, Neufing PJ, Zheng P, et al. Impaired clearance of apoptotic cardiocytes is linked to anti-SSA/Ro and -SSB/La antibodies in the pathogenesis of congenital heart block. J Clin Invest 2006;116(9):2413–22.

57. Abu-Helu RF, Dimitriou ID, Kapsogeorgou EK, et al. Induction of salivary gland epithelial cell injury in Sjögren's syndrome: in vitro assessment of T cell-derived cytokines and Fas protein expression. J Autoimmun 2001;17(2):141–53.

58. Manoussakis MN, Kapsogeorgou EK. The role of intrinsic epithelial activation in the pathogenesis of Sjögren's syndrome. J Autoimmun 2010;35(3):219–24.

59. Ohlsson M, Jonsson R, Brokstad KA. Subcellular redistribution and surface exposure of the Ro52, Ro60 and La48 autoantigens during apoptosis in human ductal epithelial cells: a possible mechanism in the pathogenesis of Sjögren's syndrome. Scand J Immunol 2002;56(5):456–69.

60. Polihronis M, Tapinos NI, Theocharis SE, et al. Modes of epithelial cell death and repair in Sjögren's syndrome (SS). Clin Exp Immunol 1998;114(3):485–90.

61. Boutjdir M, Chen L, Zhang ZH, et al. Serum and immunoglobulin G from the mother of a child with congenital heart block induce conduction abnormalities and inhibit L-type calcium channels in a rat heart model. Pediatr Res 1998; 44(1):11–9.

62. Boutjdir M, Chen L, Zhang ZH, et al. Arrhythmogenicity of IgG and anti-52-kD SSA/Ro affinity-purified antibodies from mothers of children with congenital heart block. Circ Res 1997;80(3):354–62.

63. Salomonsson S, Sonesson SE, Ottosson L, et al. Ro/SSA autoantibodies directly bind cardiomyocytes, disturb calcium homeostasis, and mediate congenital heart block. J Exp Med 2005;201(1):11–7.

64. Reed JH, Clancy RM, Purcell AW, et al. beta2-glycoprotein I and protection from anti-SSA/Ro60-associated cardiac manifestations of neonatal lupus. J Immunol 2011;187(1):520–6.

65. Briassouli P, Rifkin D, Clancy RM, et al. Binding of anti-SSA antibodies to apoptotic fetal cardiocytes stimulates urokinase plasminogen activator (uPA)/uPA receptor-dependent activation of TGF-beta and potentiates fibrosis. J Immunol 2011;187(10):5392–401.

66. Bournia VK, Vlachoyiannopoulos PG. Subgroups of Sjögren syndrome patients according to serological profiles. J Autoimmun 2012;39(1–2):15–26.

67. Martel C, Gondran G, Launay D, et al. Active immunological profile is associated with systemic Sjögren's syndrome. J Clin Immunol 2011;31(5):840–7.

68. Baldini C, Talarico R, Tzioufas AG, et al. Classification criteria for Sjögren's syndrome: a critical review. J Autoimmun 2012;39(1–2):9–14.

69. Huo AP, Lin KC, Chou CT. Predictive and prognostic value of antinuclear antibodies and rheumatoid factor in primary Sjögren's syndrome. Int J Rheum Dis 2010;13(1):39–47.

70. Kitagawa T, Shibasaki K, Toya S. Clinical significance and diagnostic usefulness of anti-centromere antibody in Sjögren's syndrome. Clin Rheumatol 2012;31(1): 105–12.

71. Peen E, Mellbye OJ, Haga HJ. IgA rheumatoid factor in primary Sjögren's syndrome. Scand J Rheumatol 2009;38(1):46–9.

72. Chung JK, Kim MK, Wee WR. Prognostic factors for the clinical severity of keratoconjunctivitis sicca in patients with Sjögren's syndrome. Br J Ophthalmol 2012; 96(2):240–5.

73. Robinson CP, Brayer J, Yamachika S, et al. Transfer of human serum IgG to non-obese diabetic Igmu null mice reveals a role for autoantibodies in the loss of secretory function of exocrine tissues in Sjögren's syndrome. Proc Natl Acad Sci U S A 1998;95(13):7538–43.

74. Passafaro D, Reina S, Sterin-Borda L, et al. Cholinergic autoantibodies from primary Sjögren's syndrome modulate submandibular gland Na+/K+-ATPase activity via prostaglandin E2 and cyclic AMP. Eur J Oral Sci 2010;118(2):131–8.

75. Reina S, Sterin-Borda L, Passafaro D, et al. Anti-M(3) muscarinic cholinergic autoantibodies from patients with primary Sjögren's syndrome trigger production of matrix metalloproteinase-3 (MMP-3) and prostaglandin E(2) (PGE(2)) from the submandibular glands. Arch Oral Biol 2011;56(5):413–20.

76. Kim N, Shin Y, Choi S, et al. Effect of antimuscarinic autoantibodies in primary Sjögren's syndrome. J Dent Res 2015;94(5):722–8.

77. Park K, Haberberger RV, Gordon TP, et al. Antibodies interfering with the type 3 muscarinic receptor pathway inhibit gastrointestinal motility and cholinergic neurotransmission in Sjögren's syndrome. Arthritis Rheum 2011;63(5):1426–34.
78. Bacman S, Berra A, Sterin-Borda L, et al. Muscarinic acetylcholine receptor antibodies as a new marker of dry eye Sjögren syndrome. Invest Ophthalmol Vis Sci 2001;42(2):321–7.
79. Cavill D, Waterman SA, Gordon TP. Failure to detect antibodies to extracellular loop peptides of the muscarinic M3 receptor in primary Sjögren's syndrome. J Rheumatol 2002;29(6):1342–4.
80. Waterman SA, Gordon TP, Rischmueller M. Inhibitory effects of muscarinic receptor autoantibodies on parasympathetic neurotransmission in Sjögren's syndrome. Arthritis Rheum 2000;43(7):1647–54.
81. Bournia VK, Diamanti KD, Vlachoyiannopoulos PG, et al. Anticentromere antibody positive Sjögren's Syndrome: a retrospective descriptive analysis. Arthritis Res Ther 2010;12(2):R47.
82. Katano K, Kawano M, Koni I, et al. Clinical and laboratory features of anticentromere antibody positive primary Sjögren's syndrome. J Rheumatol 2001;28(10): 2238–44.
83. Chan HL, Lee YS, Hong HS, et al. Anticentromere antibodies (ACA): clinical distribution and disease specificity. Clin Exp Dermatol 1994;19(4):298–302.
84. Renier G, Le Normand I, Chevailler A, et al. Anti-centromere antibodies. Study of 67 positive sera. Rev Med Interne 1992;13(6):413–4, 417–8, [in French].
85. Vlachoyiannopoulos PG, Drosos AA, Wiik A, et al. Patients with anticentromere antibodies, clinical features, diagnoses and evolution. Br J Rheumatol 1993; 32(4):297–301.
86. Moroi Y, Peebles C, Fritzler MJ, et al. Autoantibody to centromere (kinetochore) in scleroderma sera. Proc Natl Acad Sci U S A 1980;77(3):1627–31.
87. Earnshaw W, Bordwell B, Marino C, et al. Three human chromosomal autoantigens are recognized by sera from patients with anti-centromere antibodies. J Clin Invest 1986;77(2):426–30.
88. Schachna L, Wigley FM, Morris S, et al. Recognition of Granzyme B-generated autoantigen fragments in scleroderma patients with ischemic digital loss. Arthritis Rheum 2002;46(7):1873–84.
89. Pillemer SR, Casciola-Rosen L, Baum BJ, et al. Centromere protein C is a target of autoantibodies in Sjögren's syndrome and is uniformly associated with antibodies to Ro and La. J Rheumatol 2004;31(6):1121–5.
90. Gelber AC, Pillemer SR, Baum BJ, et al. Distinct recognition of antibodies to centromere proteins in primary Sjögren's syndrome compared with limited scleroderma. Ann Rheum Dis 2006;65(8):1028–32.
91. Collins K, Mitchell S, Griffiths B, et al, United Kingdom Primary Sjögren's Syndrome Registry. Potential diagnostic utility of anti-centromere antibody in primary Sjögren's syndrome in the UK. Clin Rheumatol 2012;31(7):1147–8.
92. Ramos-Casals M, Nardi N, Brito-Zeron P, et al. Atypical autoantibodies in patients with primary Sjögren syndrome: clinical characteristics and follow-up of 82 cases. Semin Arthritis Rheum 2006;35(5):312–21.
93. Barcelos F, Abreu I, Patto JV, et al. Anti-cyclic citrullinated peptide antibodies and rheumatoid factor in Sjögren's syndrome. Acta Reumatol Port 2009;34(4): 608–12.
94. Gottenberg JE, Mignot S, Nicaise-Rolland P, et al. Prevalence of anti-cyclic citrullinated peptide and anti-keratin antibodies in patients with primary Sjögren's syndrome. Ann Rheum Dis 2005;64(1):114–7.

95. Iwamoto N, Kawakami A, Tamai M, et al. Determination of the subset of Sjögren's syndrome with articular manifestations by anticyclic citrullinated peptide antibodies. J Rheumatol 2009;36(1):113–5.

96. Tobon GJ, Correa PA, Anaya JM. Anti-cyclic citrullinated peptide antibodies in patients with primary Sjögren's syndrome. Ann Rheum Dis 2005;64(5):791–2.

97. Selmi C, Meroni PL, Gershwin ME. Primary biliary cirrhosis and Sjögren's syndrome: autoimmune epithelitis. J Autoimmun 2012;39(1–2):34–42.

98. Qin Q, Wang H, Wang HZ, et al. Diagnostic accuracy of anti-alpha-fodrin antibodies for primary Sjögren's syndrome. Mod Rheumatol 2014;24(5):793–7.

99. Chen KS, Jiang MC, Li CJ, et al. Discrimination between Sjögren's and non-Sjögren's sicca syndrome by sialoscintigraphy and antibodies against alpha-fodrin and Ro/La autoantigens. J Int Med Res 2009;37(4):1088–96.

100. Nordmark G, Rorsman F, Ronnblom L, et al. Autoantibodies to alpha-fodrin in primary Sjögren's syndrome and SLE detected by an in vitro transcription and translation assay. Clin Exp Rheumatol 2003;21(1):49–56.

101. Zandbelt MM, Vogelzangs J, Van De Putte LB, et al. Anti-alpha-fodrin antibodies do not add much to the diagnosis of Sjögren's syndrome. Arthritis Res Ther 2004;6(1):R33–8.

102. Nozawa K, Ikeda K, Satoh M, et al. Autoantibody to NA14 is an independent marker primarily for Sjögren's syndrome. Front Biosci (Landmark Ed) 2009;14:3733–9.

103. Matsushita M, Matsudaira R, Ikeda K, et al. Anti-proteasome activator 28alpha is a novel anti-cytoplasmic antibody in patients with systemic lupus erythematosus and Sjögren's syndrome. Mod Rheumatol 2009;19(6):622–8.

104. Shen L, Suresh L, Lindemann M, et al. Novel autoantibodies in Sjögren's syndrome. Clin Immunol 2012;145(3):251–5.

105. Wolska N, Rybakowska P, Rasmussen A, et al. Primary Sjögren's syndrome patients with autoantibodies against TRIM38 show greater severity of disease. Arthritis Rheumatol 2016;68(3):724–9.

Genetics in Sjögren Syndrome

Tove Ragna Reksten, PhD[a,b], Christopher J. Lessard, PhD[a,c], Kathy L. Sivils, PhD[a,c,*]

KEYWORDS

- Sjögren syndrome • Genetics • RNA • Human leukocyte antigen

KEY POINTS

- The genes associated with Sjögren syndrome can be assigned to the NF-kB pathway, the IFN signaling pathway, lymphocyte signaling, and antigen presentation.
- The frequencies of risk variants show they are common with modest genetic effects, although several genes within the same pathway indicate its importance in disease pathology.
- The strongest genetic association outside the human leukocyte antigen region is in the IRF5, a gene relevant in the IFN signaling pathway and for B cell differentiation.
- Although no association has been found with the NF-kB gene itself, associations in TNFAIP3 and TNIP1 (both genome-wide significant), VCAM1 and IRAK1BP (both suggestive), point to genetic explanations for dysregulation of the NF-kB pathway in SS.

As early as 1937, Lisch suggested a hereditary link in Sjögren syndrome (SS),[1] and indeed 35% of SS patients have relatives with other autoimmune diseases.[2] Early candidate gene studies were largely based on testing risk genes identified in other autoimmune diseases.[3] Most studies have reported initial evidence for association that have not been confirmed in the larger association studies.[4] Substantial overlap has been observed in genes associated with other autoimmune diseases, such as systemic lupus erythematosus (SLE), rheumatoid arthritis (RA), inflammatory bowel disease (IBD), and psoriasis, indicating common mechanisms that lead to autoimmunity. The genetic loci implicated in autoimmunity affect cell signaling pathways, such as cytokines and cytokine receptors, and intracellular signaling pathways, such as

Disclosures: None.
[a] Arthritis and Clinical Immunology Research Program, Oklahoma Medical Research Foundation, 825 Northeast 13th Street, Oklahoma City, OK 73104, USA; [b] Broegelmann Research Laboratory, Department of Clinical Science, University of Bergen, The Laboratory Building, Haukeland University Hospital, Jonas Lies vei 87, N-5021 Bergen, Norway; [c] Department of Pathology, University of Oklahoma Health Sciences Center, 940 Stanton L. Young Boulevard, MBSB 451, Oklahoma City, OK 73104, USA
* Corresponding author. Oklahoma Medical Research Foundation, 825 Northeast 13th Street, Oklahoma City, OK 73104.
E-mail address: sivilsk@omrf.org

ubiquitination and JAK/STAT kinases, likely resulting in altered protein expression or function. Recent studies in SLE have identified a growing number of causative alleles and functional effects. For example, SLE risk variants that affect expression of RNA transcript levels have been identified for ETS1,[5] SMG7,[6] TNFAIP3,[7] and BLK.[8] Alternative mechanisms have been described, including amino acid changes that affect ligand binding (ITGAM)[9] or regulation of signaling cascades in lymphocyte activation (PTPN22).[10] With over 100 genetic variants now associated with SLE, the functional consequence of many remain elusive. More recently, large-scale genetic association studies have been conducted in SS patients. The most significant associations in SS can be grouped according to their possible functions and mechanisms of actions (**Box 1; Fig. 1**) and are the focus of this article.

ANTIGEN PRESENTATION

The human leukocyte antigen (HLA) region contains hundreds of genes that are responsible for antigen presentation and other functions in immune cells. The HLA class 1 molecules present cytosolic antigen and are expressed on all cells, whereas HLA class 2 molecules present extracellular proteins and are expressed on professional antigen presenting cells (APCs). HLA class 2 proteins convey the largest heritable predisposition for autoimmune disease (AID), including SS. The reported risk haplotypes differ slightly by phenotype and ancestral population, but a meta-analysis identified the DRB1*0301, DQA1*0501, DQB1*0201, and DRB1*03 alleles as risk factors for SS while the DQA1*0201, DQA1*0301 and DQB1*0501 alleles were protective.[11] In a recent large-scale association study of Europeans, strong associations with *HLA-DRA*, *HLA-DQB1*, and *HLA-DQA1* at the 6p21 locus were confirmed.[12] Multiple independent signals were identified, including the previously reported alleles HLA-DQA1*05:01, HLA-DQB1*02:01, and HLA-DRB*03:01. Associated variants were found to be enriched within 100 bp of binding sites for the transcription factor, RFX5, in which mutations can preclude transcription of HLA class 1 and 2 genes.[13] A study in Han Chinese identified 2 independent association signals at the 6p21.3 locus,[14] corresponding to *HLA-DRB1/HLA-DQA1* and *HLA-DPB1/COL11A2*. Breach of tolerance through abnormal antigen presentation to autoreactive T cells ovinces a key role for HLA in AID. Indeed, association with HLA disease susceptibility alleles is a common feature in AID, with shared haplotypes through the different specific alleles, and it is hypothesized that distinct alleles govern the targeting of particular autoantigens.[15] HLA class II is associated with autoantibody production in SS, as anti-Ro/SSA and anti-La/SSB are significantly increased in HLA-DQ1/HLA-DQ2 heterozygous patients,[16] but not with other clinical features,[17] and HLA DRB1*1501, but not DRB1*0301, is associated with anticyclic citrullinated antibodies (ACA).[18] Amino acid variations in the hypervariable region (HVR) of the HLA complex have been shown to affect peptide binding and presentation to T cells, and specific variation in binding pockets 7 and 9 of HLA-DRB1, altering the depth and polarity, is associated with SS in the Chinese population.[19]

Box 1
Overview of the Sjögren syndrome-associated risk genes

SS-associated risk genes are relevant in several immunologically important pathways. This simplified overview of signaling pathways and cell interactions shows how the immune cells interact and how dysregulation of genes might alter downstream effects (note that most intracellular signaling pathways are shared among the cells) (**Fig. 2**).

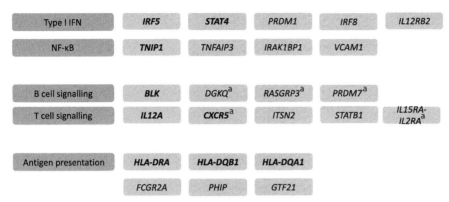

Fig. 1. Genome-wide significant ($P<5 \times 10^{-8}$) and suggestive genetic associations in Sjögren syndrome can be assigned to 4 major pathways: the IFN pathway, the NF-κB pathway, B cell signaling, and T cell signaling. The strongest genetic associations are seen for the human leukocyte antigen (HLA). **Bold** denotes genome wide significance. [a] denotes relevance in both B and T cell signaling.

THE INNATE IMMUNE RESPONSE

Three of the variants for which association with SS has been established are in genes highly relevant to innate immune responses. The most significant genetic association outside the HLA region is in the *IRF5* locus.[12] The interferon-regulatory factors (IRFs) are transcription factors that control and regulate the expression of target genes.[20] IRF5 is expressed by monocytes as a cytoplasmic protein induced by type 1 interferons (IFNs) and by Toll-like receptor (TLR) ligation[21,22] that activates transcription of several proinflammatory cytokines, including type 1 IFN, interleukin (IL)-6, IL-12, and tumor necrosis factor alpha (TNF-α).[23] A 5-bp insertion/deletion polymorphism of the *IRF5* gene was proposed to be a determinant of *IRF5* mRNA levels in PBMC, correlating with levels of IFN-induced genes.[24] However, a different model has been recently supported by studies showing the transcription factor ZBTB3, in the presence of the risk variant, exhibits increased binding to the *IRF5* promoter. This may explain the genotypically elevated expression of *IRF5*,[25] and there is evidence that the other reported risk variants alter splicing and potentially protein function.[26] Furthermore, IRF5 regulates PR domain containing 1 (Prdm1), which encodes the plasma cell maturation protein B lymphocyte-induced maturation protein 1 (Blimp-1), important for terminal B-cell differentiation[27] and Ig-secreting B1 cells. Suggestive genetic associations are seen between variants in the *PRDM1* locus and SS.[12]

A second strong genetic association is found in the gene encoding (IL12a), the p35 subunit of IL-12, with 7 variants meeting genome-wide significance and functional variants significantly influencing IL12A transcript expression.[12] IL-12, which is regulated by IRF5, is comprised of the subunit IL12p35, which is shared with IL-35 and IL12p40.[28] IL-12 is produced by myeloid cells and induces naïve CD4$^+$ T cells to differentiate into Th1 cells. Lessard and colleagues[12] further reported potential associations in the IL-12 receptor subunit B (IL12BR2), an activator of the JAK/STAT kinase pathways leading to transcription of the signal transducer and activator of transcription 4 (STAT4)[29] gene and IRF8 (also induced by IFN-γ), with further activation of IL-12 and IL-18 transcription. IL12BR2 is shared between IL-12 and IL-35, and is crucial for T helper cell 1 (T$_H$1) responses.[30]

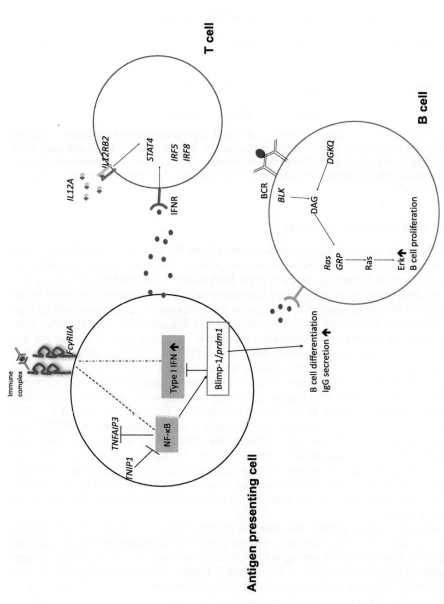

Fig. 2. Signaling pathways.

STAT4 is a well-established genetic risk factor in SS.[12,14] The activation of STAT4 by IL-12[31] provides a direct link between the cytokine receptor and gene transcription. STAT4 signaling is crucial for all biological functions of IL-12, including IFN-γ secretion[32] and CD4+ Th1 differentiation.[29] Other activators of STAT4 are IL-23[33] and IFN-α,[34,35] earning STAT4 a place in both the type 1 IFN signaling pathway and in T cell signaling. The joint effect of the 3 polymorphisms in STAT4 and IRF5 yield increased risk for SS, and the odds ratio (OR) rises from 1.43 in individuals with 2 risk alleles to 6.78 in individuals with 5 risk alleles, further stressing the importance of the type 1 IFN pathway in SS (**Box 2**).[36]

LYMPHOCYTE REGULATION AND ACTIVATION

Evidence of B and T cell abnormalities in SS is strong, and includes elevated gammaglobulins, lymphocyte retention in glands, and low peripheral lymphocyte count.[37] There is an imbalance between Th1 and Th2 cell activity in SS,[38] with a reduced ratio of Th1 to Th2.[39] T follicular helper cells (Tfh), pivotal for B cell activation and differentiation in lymphoid structures, correlate strongly with disease severity,[40] and the CD4+CXCR5+ Tfh cells are significantly increased, both locally in glands and in peripheral blood in SS patients.[41] Strong associations are seen with SNPs in the C-X-C chemokine receptor 5 (CXCR5) gene, and several regulatory elements are indicated in this region.[12] CXCR5 binds B-lymphocyte chemoattractant (BCL [also known as CXCL13]) and controls the organization of B cells in lymphoid tissue,[42] and although no significant eQTLs for CXCR5 have been demonstrated, altered protein expression or function might impact the formation of ectopic lymphoid organization in target organs in SS.

The B lymphocyte tyrosine kinase (BLK) is involved in B cell development and differentiation, transmitting signals through surface immunoglobulins, and in B cell receptor (BCR) signaling, growth arrest, and apoptosis. Variants within the shared FAM167A-BLK promoter region and in the first BLK intron have shown strong associations to SS, and variants with the potential to alter BLK expression have been identified.[12] It has been proposed that NF-κB plays a role in down-regulation of the BLK gene during plasma cell differentiation.[43]

Strong associations in TNFAIP3 interacting protein 1 (TNIP1) in the NF-κB pathway have been replicated in a European population.[12] TNIP1 encodes A20-binding inhibitor of NF-κB 1 (ABIN1), interacting with A20 to repress NF-κB.[44] A20 is encoded by the TNF-α-induced protein 3 (TNFAIP3), and represses the processing of the NF-κB

Box 2
Genetic support for the interferon signature?

The type 1 IFNs are comprised of multiple subtypes of IFN-α and 1 IFN-β. IFNs are highly pleiotropic, with antiviral, anticancer, and immunomodulatory functions.[59] Type 1 IFN signaling modulates expression of hundreds of genes,[60] and gene expression profiling in minor salivary glands (MSGs) and peripheral blood of SS patients has revealed increased expression of multiple type 1 IFN-inducible genes, a feature that is referred to as the interferon signature.[61,62] Further indications of IFN involvement are reduced IFN-producing dendritic cells (DCs) in the peripheral blood though their presence in MSGs.[63] Plasmacytoid DCs in peripheral blood are hypothesized to account for the systemic phenomenon of type 1 IFN activity,[64] and expression of TLR3 in SG epithelial cells imply that these cells may be a local source of type 1 IFNs.[65] Both IRF5 and STAT4 are genes in the IFN pathway that are strongly associated with SS, and 2 additional genes, PRDM1 and IRF8, are suggestively associated, rendering some genetic evidence for the importance of the type 1 IFN pathway. However, no direct link has been established between the genetic associations and clinical features associated with the interferon signature.

subunit p50.[44] Variants in *TNFAIP3* are strongly associated with SS in the Han Chinese population[14] and suggestively associated in Europeans. The rs2230926 SNP in *TNFAIP3* is not associated with SS; however, the rs2230926G variant is associated with lymphoma in European SS patients.[45] With suggestive genetic associations to SS in the IL-1 receptor-associated kinase 1-binding protein 1 (IRAK1BP) and potential associations for vascular cell adhesion molecule 1 (VCAM1),[12] yet another link to the NF-κB signaling pathway is established (**Box 3**). IRAK1BP is a component of the Tumor Necrosis Factor Receptor Superfamily member 1A (TNFRSF1A) signaling pathway involved in NF-κB activation,[46] and VCAM1 binds leukocyte integrins, thus recruiting lymphocytes to the site of inflammation. VCAM1 plays a role in tertiary lymphoid tissue formation,[47] and is upregulated in diseased gland tissue from SS patients.[48] Furthermore, VCAM1 is postulated to be involved in the development of vasculitis in SS patients.[49] Further suggestive associations with genes that regulate lymphocyte activity are listed in **Table 1**.

The gene most strongly associated with SS in a Northern Chinese Han population is the general transcription factor IIi (GTF2I)[14] encoding a protein involved in regulation of B and T cell activation, as well as generation of antibodies.[50,51] This association was not found in European SS patients, indicating a susceptibility locus that is race- or ethnicity-specific. Replication of the study in a Southern Chinese population confirmed the association, and found that the risk allele T of the rs117026326 SNP is slightly increased in anti-Ro/SSA-positive patients.[52] However, neither Li and colleagues nor Zheng and colleagues found any evidence that the polymorphism has any direct effect on gene expression.

OTHER GENES WITH SUGGESTIVE ASSOCIATIONS IN SJÖGREN SYNDROME

Fc receptors (FcRs) are expressed by most innate immune cells and bind immunoglobulins. FcγR bind immunoglobulin G (IgG), monomeric or aggregated, immune complexes or opsonized particles or cells. FcγRIIA, encoded by FCGR2A, is an activating receptor expressed by monocytes and macrophages, and at lower levels by dendritic cells. Polymorphisms in the FCGR2A gene modulate the affinity for some

---

Box 3
Nuclear factor kappa-B pathway and subpopulations of Sjögren syndrome

The nuclear factor kappa-B (NF-κB) family of transcription factors is comprised of 5 related factors: p50, p52, p65 (RelA), c-Rel and RelB. NF-κB has a pivotal role in host defense against stress and pathogens, the development and activation of T and B cells,[66] and in the transcription of several proinflammatory cytokine genes.[67] Dysregulation of the NF-κB signaling pathway may thus alter the inflammatory response in several ways. In SS, altered expression levels of BAFF, regulated by NF-κB, indicate a role of the transcription factor in disease pathogenesis,[68] although so far no genetic variations have been established for TNFSF13 B, the gene encoding BAFF.[69,70]

Candidate gene studies in SS patient subgroups have reported suggestive associations in several genes in the NF-κB pathway, including TNFAIP3 interacting protein 1 (TNIP1), a negative regulator of TLR- and TNF-stimulated activation of NF-κB, in anti-Ro/SSA and anti-La/SSB positive SS patients,[71] and CARD8 and TANK in germinal center (GC)-positive patients,[72] both with activation and inhibition properties of NF-κB through TNF and CD40 L mediated pathways.[73] An association with the NFKB1 gene was suggestive in a Scandinavian cohort[69] but could not be replicated in a cohort from the United Kingdom.[71]

Treatment of human salivary gland epithelial cells with anti-Ro/SSA antibodies has been shown to enhance NF-κB DNA binding and increase expression of chemokines and cytokines,[74] and the NF-κB RelA subunit is crucial for early IFN-beta expression,[75] providing a link to the IFN pathway.

Table 1
Suggestive associations with genes regulating lymphocyte activity

Gene	Full Name	Function	Association with Other AID
DGKQ	Diacylglycerol (DAG) kinase theta	Regenerate PI in the PI-cycle during cell signal transduction[a]	—
ITSN2	Intersectin 2	Regulate chlatrin-coated vesicles and TCR endocytosis[a]	—
CPEB4	Cytoplasmic polyadenylation element (CPE)-binding proteins	Translationally activate BCL-2, PI3K, IL-32 and RAS-related molecules[76]; murine CPEB4 a RORγt target gene[77]	Crohn disease[78,79]
RasGRP3	Ras guanyl-releasing protein 3	Positive Ras regulator; binds DAG, positively regulated by DAG-responsive kinases[80,81]; required for BCR-induced proliferation of B cells[82]; regulate responsiveness to TLR and IL-6 production in macrophages[83]	SLE[84]
PRDM7	PR domain containing 7	Transcription factor, possibly histone methyltransferase[a]	—
SATB1	Special AT-rich sequence binding protein 1	Chromatin recruitment and folding[85]; Th2 differentiation (IL-4, IL-5, and IL-13 induction)[86]; Treg differentiation (supressed by FoxP3)[87]; negative regulator of IL2Rα (CD25)[88]	—
IL15RA-IL2RA[b]	Interleukin receptor subunit alpha	Salivary glad NK cells critically dependent on signalling through IL-15Rα[89,90]; IL2Rα no direct contribution to signal transduction, NF-κB target gene[91]	MS, type 1 DM, SLE, RA[92–95]

Abbreviations: DM, diabetes mellitus; MS, multiple sclerosis; PI, phosphatidylinositol; RA, rheumatoid arthritis; SLE, systemic lupus erythematosus.
[a] Data from GeneCard, RefSeq.
[b] The SNP rs1323651 is located between the IL15RA and IL2RA genes.
Data from Lessard CJ, Li H, Adrianto I, et al. Variants at multiple loci implicated in both innate and adaptive immune responses are associated with Sjögren's syndrome. Nat Genet 2013;45(11):1284–92.

IgG subclasses[53] and are associated with SLE.[54] In the large European association study, a suggestive association with SS and polymorphisms in the FCGR2A gene was observed,[12] but the functional consequences remain to be elucidated.

Pleckstrin homology domain-interacting protein (PHIP) was originally identified as a protein interacting with insulin receptor substrate (IRS) 1.[55] In addition to being a modulator of the insulin receptor pathway,[56] PHIP is shown to interact with Cul4 E3 ubiquitin ligase,[57] placing this gene in the pool of SS associated loci that regulate ubiquitination, namely TNFAIP3 and TNIP1, and the Ubiquitin-Conjugating Enzyme E2E 3 (UBE2E3),[12] crucial for normal ubiquitination (from *RefSeq*).

Several additional genes that do not belong to any of the outlined pathways were identified as suggestively associated with SS. These include genes involved in RNA binding (CPEB4, ATXN2), noncoding and micro-RNA (TP53TG1, MIR1208), the estrogen-induced ABHD6 locus, and genes important for cell growth and proliferation (DOCK1-NPS, TPD52L2).[12]

Finally, a new genetic explanation has been suggested to elucidate the gender bias observed in female-predominant autoimmune diseases. The prevalence of triple X syndrome (47,XXX) is approximately 1 in 1000 in the general public, but 1 in 344 in SS patients, estimating the prevalence of SS in women with triple X syndrome (47,XXX) at 2.9 times higher than in 46,XX women.[58] In addition, unpublished data show that 47,XXY is increased among men with SS (Harris VM, et al, 2016).

REFERENCES

1. Lisch K. Über hereditäres Vorkommen des mit Keratoconjunctivitis sicca verbundenen Sjögrenschen Symptomenkomplexes. Arch f Augenh 1937;110:357–64.
2. Reveille JD, Wilson RW, Provost TT, et al. Primary Sjögren's syndrome and other autoimmune diseases in families. Prevalence and immunogenetic studies in six kindreds. Ann Intern Med 1984;101(6):748–56.
3. Ice JA, Li H, Adrianto I, et al. Genetics of Sjögren's syndrome in the genome-wide association era. J Autoimmun 2012;39(1–2):57–63.
4. Nezos A, Mavragani CP. Contribution of genetic factors to Sjögren's syndrome and Sjögren's syndrome related lymphomagenesis. J Immunol Res 2015; 2015(11):754825–912.
5. Lu X, Zoller EE, Weirauch MT, et al. Lupus risk variant increases pSTAT1 Binding and Decreases ETS1 Expression. Am J Hum Genet 2015;96(5):731–9.
6. Deng Y, Zhao J, Sakurai D, et al. Decreased SMG7 expression associates with lupus-risk variants and elevated antinuclear antibody production. Ann Rheum Dis 2016. http://dx.doi.org/10.1136/annrheumdis-2015-208441.
7. Adrianto I, Wang S, Wiley GB, et al. Association of two independent functional risk haplotypes in TNIP1 with systemic lupus erythematosus. Arthritis Rheum 2012; 64(11):3695–705.
8. Guthridge JM, Lu R, Sun H, et al. Two functional lupus-associated BLK promoter variants control cell-type- and developmental-stage-specific transcription. Am J Hum Genet 2014;94(4):586–98.
9. Fagerholm SC, MacPherson M, James MJ, et al. The CD11b-integrin (ITGAM) and systemic lupus erythematosus. Lupus 2013;22(7):657–63.
10. Wang Y, Ewart D, Crabtree JN, et al. PTPN22 Variant R620W Is Associated With Reduced Toll-like Receptor 7-Induced Type I Interferon in Systemic Lupus Erythematosus. Arthritis Rheum 2015;67(9):2403–14.
11. Cruz-Tapias P, Rojas-Villarraga A, Maier-Moore S, et al. HLA and Sjögren's syndrome susceptibility. A meta-analysis of worldwide studies. Autoimmun Rev 2012;11(4):281–7.
12. Lessard CJ, Li H, Adrianto I, et al. Variants at multiple loci implicated in both innate and adaptive immune responses are associated with Sjögren's syndrome. Nat Genet 2013;45(11):1284–92.
13. Nekrep N, Jabrane-Ferrat N, Wolf HM, et al. Mutation in a winged-helix DNA-binding motif causes atypical bare lymphocyte syndrome. Nat Immunol 2002;3(11):1075–81.
14. Li Y, Zhang K, Chen H, et al. A genome-wide association study in Han Chinese identifies a susceptibility locus for primary Sjögren's syndrome at 7q11.23. Nat Genet 2013;45(11):1361–5.
15. Fernando MMA, Stevens CR, Walsh EC, et al. Defining the role of the MHC in autoimmunity: a review and pooled analysis. PLoS Genet 2008;4(4):e1000024.

16. Harley JB, Reichlin M, Arnett FC, et al. Gene interaction at HLA-DQ enhances auto-antibody production in primary Sjögren's syndrome. Science 1986;232(4754): 1145–7.
17. Gottenberg J-E, Busson M, Loiscau P, et al. In primary Sjögren's syndrome, HLA class II is associated exclusively with autoantibody production and spreading of the autoimmune response. Arthritis Rheum 2003;48(8):2240–5.
18. Mohammed K, Pope J, Le Riche N, et al. Association of severe inflammatory polyarthritis in primary Sjögren's syndrome: clinical, serologic, and HLA analysis. J Rheumatol 2009;36(9):1937–42.
19. Huang R, Yin J, Chen Y, et al. The amino acid variation within the binding pocket 7 and 9 of HLA-DRB1 molecules are associated with primary Sjögren's syndrome. J Autoimmun 2015;57:53–9.
20. Taniguchi T, Ogasawara K, Takaoka A, et al. IRF family of transcription factors as regulators of host defense. Annu Rev Immunol 2001;19(1):623–55.
21. Takaoka A, Yanai H, Kondo S, et al. Integral role of IRF-5 in the gene induction programme activated by Toll-like receptors. Nature 2005;434(7030):243–9.
22. Honda K, Yanai H, Mizutani T, et al. Role of a transductional-transcriptional pro-cessor complex involving MyD88 and IRF-7 in Toll-like receptor signaling. Proc Natl Acad Sci U S A 2004;101(43):15416–21.
23. Honda K, Taniguchi T. IRFs: master regulators of signaling by Toll-like receptors and cytosolic pattern-recognition receptors. Nat Rev Immunol 2006;6(9):644–58.
24. Miceli-Richard C, Gestermann N, Ittah M, et al. The CGGGG insertion/deletion polymorphism of the IRF5 promoter is a strong risk factor for primary Sjögren's syndrome. Arthritis Rheum 2009;60(7):1991–7.
25. Kottyan LC, Zoller EE, Bene J, et al. The IRF5-TNPO3 association with systemic lupus erythematosus has two components that other autoimmune disorders variably share. Hum Mol Genet 2015;24(2):582–96.
26. Graham RR, Kyogoku C, Sigurdsson S, et al. Three functional variants of IFN regulatory factor 5 (IRF5) define risk and protective haplotypes for human lupus. Proc Natl Acad Sci U S A 2007;104(16):6758–63.
27. Lien C, Fang C-M, Huso D, et al. Critical role of IRF-5 in regulation of B-cell differentiation. Proc Natl Acad Sci U S A 2010;107(10):4664–8.
28. Sun L, He C, Nair L, et al. Interleukin 12 (IL-12) family cytokines: Role in immune pathogenesis and treatment of CNS autoimmune disease. Cytokine 2015;75(2): 249–55.
29. Nishikomori R, Usui T, Wu C-Y, et al. Activated STAT4 has an essential role in Th1 differentiation and proliferation that is independent of its role in the maintenance of IL-12R beta 2 chain expression and signaling. J Immunol 2002;169(8):4388–98.
30. Giese NA, Gabriele L, Doherty TM, et al. Interferon (IFN) consensus sequence-binding protein, a transcription factor of the IFN regulatory factor family, regulates immune responses in vivo through control of interleukin 12 expression. J Exp Med 1997;186(9):1535–46.
31. Leonard WJ, O'Shea JJ. Jaks and STATs: biological implications. Annu Rev Immunol 1998;16(1):293–322.
32. Lawless VA, Zhang S, Ozes ON, et al. Stat4 regulates multiple components of IFN-gamma-inducing signaling pathways. J Immunol 2000;165(12):6803–8.
33. Mathur AN, Chang H-C, Zisoulis DG, et al. Stat3 and Stat4 direct development of IL-17-secreting Th cells. J Immunol 2007;178(8):4901–7.
34. Cho SS, Bacon CM, Sudarshan C, et al. Activation of STAT4 by IL-12 and IFN-alpha: evidence for the involvement of ligand-induced tyrosine and serine phosphorylation. J Immunol 1996;157(11):4781–9.

35. Matikainen S, Paananen A, Miettinen M, et al. IFN-alpha and IL-18 synergistically enhance IFN-gamma production in human NK cells: differential regulation of Stat4 activation and IFN-gamma gene expression by IFN-alpha and IL-12. Eur J Immunol 2001;31(7):2236–45.

36. Nordmark G, Kristjansdottir G, Theander E, et al. Additive effects of the major risk alleles of IRF5 and STAT4 in primary Sjögren's syndrome. Genes Immun 2009; 10(1):68–76.

37. Fox RI, Howell FV, Bone RC, et al. Primary Sjogren syndrome: clinical and immunopathologic features. Semin Arthritis Rheum 1984;14(2):77–105.

38. van Woerkom JM. Salivary gland and peripheral blood T helper 1 and 2 cell activity in Sjogren"s syndrome compared with non-Sjogren"s sicca syndrome. Ann Rheum Dis 2005;64(10):1474–9.

39. Kohriyama K, Katayama Y. Disproportion of helper T cell subsets in peripheral blood of patients with primary Sjögren's syndrome. Autoimmunity 2000;32(1):67–72.

40. Szabo K, Papp G, Barath S, et al. Follicular helper T cells may play an important role in the severity of primary Sjögren's syndrome. Clin Immunol 2013;147(2):95–104.

41. Jin L, Yu D, Li X, et al. CD4+CXCR5+ follicular helper T cells in salivary gland promote B cells maturation in patients with primary Sjögren's syndrome. Int J Clin Exp Pathol 2014;7(5):1988–96.

42. Ansel KM, Ngo VN, Hyman PL, et al. A chemokine-driven positive feedback loop organizes lymphoid follicles. Nature 2000;406(6793):309–14.

43. Zwollo P, Rao S, Wallin JJ, et al. The transcription factor NF-kappaB/p50 interacts with the blk gene during B cell activation. J Biol Chem 1998;273(29):18647–55.

44. Ramirez VP, Gurevich I, Aneskievich BJ. Emerging roles for TNIP1 in regulating post-receptor signaling. Cytokine Growth Factor Rev 2012;23(3):109–18.

45. Nocturne G, Tarn J, Boudaoud S, et al. Germline variation of TNFAIP3 in primary Sjögren's syndrome-associated lymphoma. Ann Rheum Dis 2015. http://dx.doi.org/10.1136/annrheumdis-2015-207731.

46. Stelzer G, Dalah I, Stein TI, et al. In-silico human genomics with GeneCards. Hum Genomics 2011;5(6):709–17.

47. Neyt K, Perros F, GeurtsvanKessel CH, et al. Tertiary lymphoid organs in infection and autoimmunity. Trends Immunol 2012;33(6):297–305.

48. Saito I, Terauchi K, Shimuta M, et al. Expression of cell adhesion molecules in the salivary and lacrimal glands of Sjogren's syndrome. J Clin Lab Anal 1993;7(3):180–7.

49. Turkcapar N, Sak SD, Saatci M, et al. Vasculitis and expression of vascular cell adhesion molecule-1, intercellular adhesion molecule-1, and E-selectin in salivary glands of patients with Sjögren's syndrome. J Rheumatol 2005;32(6):1063–70.

50. Sacristán C, Schattgen SA, Berg LJ, et al. Characterization of a novel interaction between transcription factor TFII-I and the inducible tyrosine kinase in T cells. Eur J Immunol 2009;39(9):2584–95.

51. Yang W, Desiderio S. BAP-135, a target for Bruton's tyrosine kinase in response to B cell receptor engagement. Proc Natl Acad Sci U S A 1997;94(2):604–9.

52. Zheng J, Huang R, Huang Q, et al. The GTF2I rs117026326 polymorphism is associated with anti-SSA-positive primary Sjögren's syndrome. Rheumatology (Oxford) 2015;54(3):562–4.

53. Bruhns P, Iannascoli B, England P, et al. Specificity and affinity of human Fcgamma receptors and their polymorphic variants for human IgG subclasses. Blood 2009;113(16):3716–25.

54. Li X, Ptacek TS, Brown EE, et al. Fcgamma receptors: structure, function and role as genetic risk factors in SLE. Genes Immun 2009;10(5):380–9.

55. Farhang-Fallah J, Randhawa VK, Nimnual A, et al. The pleckstrin homology (PH) domain-interacting protein couples the insulin receptor substrate 1 PH domain to insulin signaling pathways leading to mitogenesis and GLUT4 translocation. Mol Cell Biol 2002;22(20):7325–36.

56. Farhang-Fallah J, Yin X, Trentin G, et al. Cloning and characterization of PHIP, a novel insulin receptor substrate-1 pleckstrin homology domain interacting protein. J Biol Chem 2000;275(51):40492–7.

57. Jin J, Arias EE, Chen J, et al. A family of diverse Cul4-Ddb1-interacting proteins includes Cdt2, which is required for S phase destruction of the replication factor Cdt1. Mol Cell 2006;23(5):709–21.

58. Liu K, Kurien BT, Zimmerman SL, et al. X chromosome dose and sex bias in autoimmune diseases: increased 47,XXX in systemic lupus erythematosus and Sjögren's syndrome. Arthritis Rheum 2015. http://dx.doi.org/10.1002/art.39560.

59. Stark GR. How cells respond to interferons revisited: from early history to current complexity. Cytokine Growth Factor Rev 2007;18(5–6):419–23.

60. Der SD, Zhou A, Williams BR, et al. Identification of genes differentially regulated by interferon alpha, beta, or gamma using oligonucleotide arrays. Proc Natl Acad Sci U S A 1998;95(26):15623–8.

61. Hjelmervik TOR, Petersen K, Jonassen I, et al. Gene expression profiling of minor salivary glands clearly distinguishes primary Sjögren's syndrome patients from healthy control subjects. Arthritis Rheum 2005;52(5):1534–44.

62. Emamian ES, Leon JM, Lessard CJ, et al. Peripheral blood gene expression profiling in Sjögren's syndrome. Genes Immun 2009;10(4):285–96.

63. Vogelsang P, Brun JG, Oijordsbakken G, et al. Levels of plasmacytoid dendritic cells and type-2 myeloid dendritic cells are reduced in peripheral blood of patients with primary Sjogren's syndrome. Ann Rheum Dis 2010;69(6):1235–8.

64. Wildenberg ME, van Helden-Meeuwsen CG, van de Merwe JP, et al. Systemic increase in type I interferon activity in Sjögren's syndrome: a putative role for plasmacytoid dendritic cells. Eur J Immunol 2008;38(7):2024–33.

65. Spachidou MP, Bourazopoulou E, Maratheftis CI, et al. Expression of functional Toll-like receptors by salivary gland epithelial cells: increased mRNA expression in cells derived from patients with primary Sjögren's syndrome. Clin Exp Immunol 2007;147(3):497–503.

66. Siebenlist U, Brown K, Claudio E. Control of lymphocyte development by nuclear factor-kappaB. Nat Rev Immunol 2005;5(6):435–45.

67. Hayden MS, Ghosh S. NF-κB in immunobiology. Cell Res 2011;21(2):223–44.

68. Groom J, Kalled SL, Cutler AH, et al. Association of BAFF/BLyS overexpression and altered B cell differentiation with Sjögren's syndrome. J Clin Invest 2002; 109(1):59–68.

69. Nordmark G, Kristjansdottir G, Theander E, et al. Association of EBF1, FAM167A(C8orf13)-BLK and TNFSF4 gene variants with primary Sjögren's syndrome. Genes Immun 2010;12(2):1–10.

70. Gottenberg J-E, Sellam J, Ittah M, et al. No evidence for an association between the -871 T/C promoter polymorphism in the B-cell-activating factor gene and primary Sjögren's syndrome. Arthritis Res Ther 2006;8(1):R30.

71. Nordmark G, Wang C, Vasaitis L, et al. Association of genes in the NF-κB pathway with antibody-positive primary Sjögren's syndrome. Scand J Immunol 2013;78(5):447–54.

72. Reksten TR, Johnsen SJA, Jonsson MV, et al. Genetic associations to germinal centre formation in primary Sjogren's syndrome. Ann Rheum Dis 2014;73(6):1253–8.

73. Cheng G, Baltimore D. TANK, a co-inducer with TRAF2 of TNF- and CD 40L-mediated NF-kappaB activation. Genes Dev 1996;10(8):963–73.

74. Lisi S, Sisto M, Lofrumento DD, et al. Sjögren's syndrome autoantibodies provoke changes in gene expression profiles of inflammatory cytokines triggering a pathway involving TACE/NF-kappa. Lab Invest 2011;92(4):615–24.

75. Wang J, Basagoudanavar SH, Wang X, et al. NF-kappa B RelA subunit is crucial for early IFN-beta expression and resistance to RNA virus replication. J Immunol 2010;185(3):1720–9.

76. Ortiz-Zapater E, Pineda D, nez-Bosch NMI, et al. Key contribution of CPEB4-mediated translational control to cancer progression. Nat Med 2011; 18(1):83–90.

77. Xi H, Schwartz R, Engel I, et al. Interplay between RORgammat, Egr3, and E proteins controls proliferation in response to pre-TCR signals. Immunity 2006;24(6):813–26.

78. Franke A, McGovern DPB, Barrett JC, et al. Genome-wide meta-analysis increases to 71 the number of confirmed Crohn's disease susceptibility loci. Nat Genet 2010;42(12):1118–25.

79. Jostins L, Ripke S, Weersma RK, et al. Host-microbe interactions have shaped the genetic architecture of inflammatory bowel disease. Nature 2012;491(7422):119–24.

80. Lorenzo PS, Kung JW, Bottorff DA, et al. Phorbol esters modulate the Ras exchange factor RasGRP3. Cancer Res 2001;61(3):943–9.

81. Teixeira C, Stang SL, Zheng Y, et al. Integration of DAG signaling systems mediated by PKC-dependent phosphorylation of RasGRP3. Blood 2003;102(4):1414–20.

82. Coughlin JJ, Stang SL, Dower NA, et al. RasGRP1 and RasGRP3 regulate B cell proliferation by facilitating B cell receptor-Ras signaling. J Immunol 2005;175(11): 7179–84.

83. Tang S, Chen T, Yu Z, et al. RasGRP3 limits Toll-like receptor-triggered inflammatory response in macrophages by activating Rap1 small GTPase. Nat Commun 2014;5:4657.

84. Molineros JE, Chua KH, Sun C, et al. Evaluation of SLE Susceptibility Genes in Malaysians. Autoimmune Dis 2014;2014(10):305436–8.

85. Yasui D, Miyano M, Cai S, et al. SATB1 targets chromatin remodeling to regulate genes over long distances. Nature 2002;419(6907):641–5.

86. Cai S, Lee CC, Kohwi-Shigematsu T. SATB1 packages densely looped, transcriptionally active chromatin for coordinated expression of cytokine genes. Nat Genet 2006;38(11):1278–88.

87. Beyer M, Thabet Y, Müller R-U, et al. Repression of the genome organizer SATB1 in regulatory T cells is required for suppressive function and inhibition of effector differentiation. Nat Immunol 2011;12(9):898–907.

88. Kumar PP, Purbey PK, Ravi DS, et al. Displacement of SATB1-bound histone deacetylase 1 corepressor by the human immunodeficiency virus type 1 transactivator induces expression of interleukin-2 and its receptor in T cells. Mol Cell Biol 2005;25(5):1620–33.

89. Tessmer MS, Reilly EC, Brossay L. Salivary gland NK cells are phenotypically and functionally unique. Plos Pathog 2011;7(1):e1001254.

90. Cortez VS, Fuchs A, Cella M, et al. Cutting edge: Salivary gland NK cells develop independently of Nfil3 in steady-state. J Immunol 2014;192(10):4487–91.

91. Ballard DW, Böhnlein E, Lowenthal JW, et al. HTLV-I tax induces cellular proteins that activate the kappa B element in the IL-2 receptor alpha gene. Science 1988; 241(4873):1652–5.

92. Babron M-C, Perdry H, Handel AE, et al. Determination of the real effect of genes identified in GWAS: the example of IL2RA in multiple sclerosis. Eur J Hum Genet 2012;20(3):321–5.
93. Garg G, Tyler JR, Yang JHM, et al. Type 1 diabetes-associated IL2RA variation lowers IL-2 signaling and contributes to diminished CD4+CD25+ regulatory T cell function. J Immunol 2012;188(9):4644–53.
94. Elghzaly AA, Metwally SS, El-Chennawi FA, et al. IRF5, PTPN22, CD28, IL2RA, KIF5A, BLK and TNFAIP3 genes polymorphisms and lupus susceptibility in a cohort from the Egypt Delta; relation to other ethnic groups. Hum Immunol 2015;76(7):525–31.
95. van Steenbergen HW, van Nies JAB, Ruyssen-Witrand A, et al. IL2RA is associated with persistence of rheumatoid arthritis. Arthritis Res Ther 2015;17(1):244.

The Proteomics of Saliva in Sjögren's Syndrome

Stergios Katsiougiannis, PhD, David T.W. Wong, DMD, DMSc*

KEYWORDS

- Sjögren's syndrome • Saliva • Proteomics • Biomarkers • Saliva diagnostics

KEY POINTS

- Sjögren's syndrome (SS) saliva proteome analysis reveals a unique expression profile.
- Major classification biomarkers of SS are present in saliva, including anti-Ro/SSA and anti-La/SSB.
- Prevalidation studies suggest salivary autoantibodies as strong biomarker candidates in SS.
- Further clinical validation of the verified and prevalidated proteomic signatures is needed in independent multicenter validation cohorts.

INTRODUCTION

Primary SS (pSS) is characterized by chronic dysfunction and destruction of exocrine glands, in particular the salivary and lacrimal glands, leading to persistent dryness of the mouth and eyes.[1] Due to the direct involvement of those glands in the pathophysiology of the disease, saliva and tears are thought to reflect the glandular dysfunction and destruction. Saliva and tears drain the main targets of autoimmune response, which in the case of pSS are the salivary and lacrimal glands.

Saliva presents obvious advantages in terms of accessibility and unstimulated secretion, hence, ease of collection. Although primarily considered an indispensable element of early digestion, saliva is a heterogeneous biofluid comprised of

Disclosure: D.T.W. Wong is cofounder of RNAmeTRIX Inc, a molecular diagnostic company. He holds equity in RNAmeTRIX and serves as a company Director and Scientific Advisor. The University of California also holds equity in RNAmeTRIX. Intellectual property that D.T.W. Wong invented and that was patented by the University of California has been licensed to RNAmeTRIX.

Supported by research grants to D.T.W. Wong: National Institute of Dental and Craniofacial Research, U01DE017593, and to S. Katsiougiannis: Hirshberg Foundation Seed grant 2015.

Center for Oral/Head and Neck Oncology Research, Division of Oral Biology, School of Dentistry, UCLA, 10833 Le Conte Avenue, CHS 73-034, Los Angeles, CA 90095, USA

* Corresponding author. Center for Oral/Head and Neck Oncology Research, School of Dentistry, 10833 Le Conte Avenue, CHS 73-034, Los Angeles, CA 90095.

E-mail address: dtww@ucla.edu

biomolecules and omics constituents, which may become altered in response to various diseases, including pSS. The advancements of high-throughput technologies and analytical techniques have made saliva proteomics an ideal tool to study the underlying pSS glandular autoimmune exocrinopathy. In recent years, scientific effort has been undertaken for the purpose of evaluating saliva proteome to diagnose, monitor, or prognosticate pSS. The results from these studies are encouraging; thus, saliva has been emerged as a novel and promising biofluid for the discovery of definitive disease-specific biomarkers for pSS with potential clinical and translational impact.[2,3]

This discussion begins by exploring the production, secretion and composition of saliva. Next, the proteomics of saliva in the context of pSS are delved into by describing several studies conducted from different groups including the authors'. Last, potential pitfalls are addressed and promising topics highlighted for the near future of saliva-proteome research in pSS.

SALIVA: PRODUCTION AND SECRETION

Saliva is produced by several salivary glands located around the oral cavity, including the parotid, submandibular, sublingual, and minor salivary glands and the posterior deep lingual glands (von Ebner glands). Salivary glands are comprised of clustered acinar cells called acini, which concertedly produce approximately 500 mL to 1500 mL of saliva daily.[4]

Two categories of acinar cells are found in the salivary glands: (1) serous cells (most commonly found in the parotid gland), which secrete a nonviscous watery product, and (2) mucous cells (predominant in the sublingual gland), which secrete a mucous-like product of high viscosity. The solution produced by these cells contains electrolytes, mucins, and enzymes, which subsequently flow into collecting tubes, where their composition can be further altered by the reabsorption of specific molecules before release into the mouth as saliva.

COMPOSITION

Saliva is a clear, slightly acidic, hypotonic fluid, which is continuously secreted and is predominantly composed of water (99.5%). The remaining 0.5% is comprised of inorganic ions, including sodium, chloride, potassium, and calcium along with organic components, such as proteins, amino acids, antibodies, hormones, enzymes, lipids and cytokines, among many others.[5] In addition, recent studies have shown that saliva actually contains a variety of genomic, transcriptomic, proteomic, microbiologic, and immunologic analytes[6–9] that may be capable of identifying both local and systemic disorders in afflicted individuals. Therefore, saliva is now the focal point of multiple investigations aimed at establishing oral fluids as the preferred diagnostic medium.

In 2004 the National Institute of Dental and Craniofacial Research provided funding to 3 research groups comprising the Saliva Proteome Consortium, in an effort to identify and catalog the human saliva proteome, including saliva proteins as well as their structurally modified forms (eg, glycosylated and phosphorylated). These studies revealed the salivary proteome as a sizeable collection of up to 1166 protein molecules—914 in parotid saliva and 917 in submandibular/sublingual saliva.[10] A majority of these proteins are synthesized and secreted into the oral cavity by the acinar cells of the salivary glands. In consideration, a high proportion of proteins that are found in plasma and/or tears are also present in saliva along with unique components.[8,10–12] The proteins identified are involved in numerous molecular processes, ranging from structural functions to enzymatic and catalytic activities, with a majority of them mapped to the extracellular and secretory compartments.

FUNCTION

Saliva plays a key role in maintaining the oral health and homeostasis, by lubricating and moistening the oral tissues to aid in swallowing, chewing, speech, and taste.[13] Saliva also has a critical role in initiating and facilitating digestion. In addition, maintenance of oral health largely depends on saliva's cleansing actions and intrinsic antipathogenic characteristics.[14]

SALIVA FOR BIOMARKER DISCOVERY IN PRIMARY SJÖGREN SYNDROME
An Attractive Biofluid

The revelation that saliva is comprised of analytes capable of reflecting health status presents a significant translation potential. In considering the simplicity of saliva collection and its potential as a diagnostic medium, oral fluids have rapidly become the focus of investigation for several disease biomarkers. In that sense, saliva is widely recognized as an attractive biofluid for study of pSS, featuring several undisputable advantages over blood, the most important that it can be obtained using noninvasive techniques. As a clinical tool, saliva can be easily collected, stored, and shipped compared with serum. More importantly, for patients, the noninvasive collection techniques significantly reduce anxiety and discomfort and make procurement of repeated collections a cost-effective approach for longitudinal monitoring.[8,15,16]

Challenges

Although saliva exerts several compelling advantages over serum and other invasively collected biofluids, there are challenges that need to be overcome.[17] Unlike blood, saliva proteome seems sensitive to degradation and research has been carried out to minimize those processes. Hence, a major challenge is to collect and store saliva under conditions that prevent proteolysis, degradation, or dephosphorylation. The authors have shown that collection of saliva into ice-cold tubes, addition of protease inhibitors, and storage immediately at -80°C result in minimal proteolysis.[18] Another critical step for proper saliva proteomic analysis is the removal of the mucins. These proteins are responsible for the "sticky" appearance of saliva and might interact with standard immunologic assays. Mucins removal can be achieved either by centrifugation or by using special filter-containing collection devices.

Immunologic Proteins in Saliva

One of the current criteria used for diagnosis of pSS is serum positivity for anti-Ro/SSA and/or anti-La/SSB.[19] Studies from different groups have demonstrated the presence of these 2 autoantibodies in whole and parotid saliva collected from pSS patients.[20–23] This finding is of fundamental importance for pSS because it provides evidence that oral fluids are capable of reflecting the autoantibody load, thus presenting an alternative, noninvasive procedure for the diagnosis of the disease. Other autoantibodies that have been described in saliva are anti-mAChR, anti-spectrin, and rheumatoid factor.[24–27] In an attempt not only to discover but also validate potential autoantibody biomarkers in saliva, the authors' laboratory has identified 24 potential autoantibodies that can discriminate patients with SS from both patients with systemic lupus erythematosus and healthy individuals. Four of these saliva autoantibodies, namely anti-transglutaminase, anti-histone, anti-Ro/SSA, and anti-La/SSB, were further successfully validated in independent SS, systemic lupus erythematosus, and healthy control subjects.[22] Hence, saliva autoantibodies seem promising biomarkers to be used in a clinical setting.

A few studies have reported saliva cytokines in the context of pSS. Data from these reports congruently show significantly higher levels of T_H1, T_H2, and T_H17 cytokines in saliva of pSS patients.[28–31] The lack of appropriate controls in a majority of these studies, non-SS sicca patients, however, does not allow a definitive conclusion regarding the specificity of these salivary cytokines to discriminate pSS from non-SS sicca subjects. Kang and colleagues[28] found that salivary T_H1/T_H2 ratios, represented by interferon-γ/interleukin (IL)-4 and by tumor necrosis factor α/IL-4 ratios, were features that most differentiated SS and non-SS sicca and were correlated with the clinical parameters of SS.

To conclude, the available data indicate that immunologic proteins, including the major pSS-related autoantibodies and cytokines, can be detected in saliva and their levels are significantly increased in patients suffering from pSS. These findings, although not independently validated in large clinical cohorts, confirm that saliva is capable of reflecting the autoimmune exocrinopathy in pSS.

Salivary Proteomics for Primary Sjögren Syndrome Diagnosis

Because saliva is the product of salivary glands, the primary targets of the autoimmune response in pSS, it is believed that this secreted fluid can directly mirror the glands' pathophysiology. To analyze the proteomic content of saliva, scientists often use traditional techniques, including liquid chromatography, gel and capillary electrophoresis, nuclear magnetic resonance, mass spectrography, and immunoassays.[32] More contemporary methods, however, including immune-response protoarrays and 2-D electrophoresis (2DE) coupled with mass spectrography, are also used and have allowed investigators to analyze several salivary analytes.[22,33,34] The development of emerging high-throughput proteomic approaches allows the investigation of the whole and gland-specific protein composition.

The main goal of these studies has been the discovery, verification, and validation of a panel of protein biomarkers so that they can be used in early detection of pSS. Such approaches have highlighted distinct protein patterns characteristic of pSS.[2,3,33–39] These protein signatures mostly comprise secretory proteins, enzymes, calcium-binding proteins, and abundantly expressed immune-related molecules, such as β_2-microglobulin.[33,35,37,39] Other protein molecules that have received particular attention include cathepsin-D, α-enolase, cystatins, defensins, and Ig γ light chain. Collectively, these studies have presented evidence that inflammatory phase proteins are elevated in saliva from pSS patients and this finding correlates with the chronic autoimmune inflammation of the salivary glands in pSS. Similarly, the increased expression of salivary β_2-microglobulin, Ig κ light chain, and Ig γ light chain was attributed to B-cell activation in the periphery. In an effort to catalog salivary biomarkers according to their biological pathways, a recent study showed that SS-associated salivary proteome seems profoundly altered with respect to several aspects of immunity, immune cell differentiation, and tissue homeostasis.[40] The congruency between the proteomic signatures identified in this study and the hallmarks of salivary gland pathology in pSS greatly supports that salivary proteome reflects the biologic state of the glands. Collectively, these data indicate that saliva has the capability of revealing changes in the biologic state of the salivary glands and proteomic approaches seem a promising tool for improving early diagnosis of pSS.

Prognostic Biomarkers of Lymphoma in Primary Sjögren Syndrome

Considering the lack of well-validated prediction biomarkers,[41,42] saliva might be a significant pool of candidate molecules for early identification of pSS patients at higher risk for developing mucosa-associated lymphoid tissue (MALT) lymphoma. The authors' group has performed a proteomic and transcriptomic analysis of human parotid glands from patients with pSS and patients with pSS and MALT lymphoma.[43] This study revealed that 70 proteins were up-regulated in SS/MALT lymphoma samples compared with both non–SS control and pSS samples. Intriguingly, 45% of the up-regulated proteins had an mRNA transcript (gene-expression level) that was concordantly differentially expressed. Most of the proteins with up-regulated levels in pSS/MALT lymphoma were related to signal transduction, gene regulation, apoptosis, and the immune response. Among these targets, a few have previously been linked to lymphoma, and, in particular, 2 cancer-related proteins, Rho-GDP dissociation inhibitor and cyclophilin A, are of biologic significance.

In another proteomic approach to analyze whole saliva from pSS and pSS/MALT lymphoma patients, Baldini and colleagues[44] showed several qualitative and quantitative modifications in the expression of putative albumin, immunoglobulin J chain, Ig kappa chain C region, α_1-antitrypsin, haptoglobin, and Ig α_1-chain C region. These studies suggest that clinical and functional changes of the salivary glands driven by lymphoproliferative processes might be reflected in patients' whole saliva, providing further insights into the molecular mechanisms of pSS and pSS/MALT lymphoma. Reasonably, once validated and confirmed, the identified protein candidates could be translated into early prognostic biomarkers for non-Hodgkin lymphoma–susceptible pSS patients.

SUMMARY

In the past few years, saliva proteomics has emerged as a promising source for the discovery of pSS biomarkers, for use in diagnosis, classification, and/or predicting the prognosis of patients with pSS. Saliva is the obvious pool of these biomarkers, because it is directly and constantly secreted by the primarily affected exocrine glands. Thus, the translation of basic research findings into clinical practice is of great importance. In this regard, effort is been undertaken by multiple research groups for the definitive validation of salivary biomarkers in large, independent multicenter cohorts. These ongoing studies will validate the previously identified and verified salivary proteins and strengthen their potential as biomarkers for pSS. Furthermore, the correlation of salivary biomarker profiles with salivary function and clinical diseases would help in the stratification of pSS patients, which is required for their proper treatment. The dependency on lip biopsy hampers efficient early assessment of an individual with suspicious pSS; thus, the development of such biomarkers has the potential to resolve several challenges that hinder effective on-time evaluation and diagnosis. In conclusion, saliva proteomics have potential for the development of biomarkers and for the identification of pathogenic pathways underlying the different subsets of pSS, leading to the development of new treatment strategies (**Table 1**).

Table 1
Salivary autoantibodies in primary Sjögren syndrome

Salivary Autoantibodies	Saliva Sample	Authors, y
IgA rheumatoid factor, IgM rheumatoid factor	Whole saliva	Dunne et al,[24] 1979
Anti-Ro/SSA, anti-La/SSB	Whole saliva	Ben-Chetrit et al,[23] 1993
IgA rheumatoid factor	Whole saliva	Markusse et al,[21] 1993
Anti-spectrin	Parotid Saliva	Moody et al,[26] 2001
Anti-Ro52, anti-Ro60	Whole saliva	Ching et al,[20] 2011
Anti-Ro/SSA, anti-La/SSB, Anti-histone, anti-transglutaminase	Whole saliva	Hu et al,[22] 2011
Anti-M_3 mAChR IgA	Whole saliva	Berra et al,[25] 2002
Anti-M_3 mAChR-220	Whole saliva	He et al,[27] 2012

REFERENCES

1. Manoussakis MN, Moutsopoulos HM. Sjogren's syndrome: autoimmune epithelitis. Baillieres Best Pract Res Clin Rheumatol 2000;14:73–95.
2. Giusti L, Baldini C, Bazzichi L, et al. Proteomic diagnosis of Sjogren's syndrome. Expert Rev Proteomics 2007;4:757–67.
3. Hu S, Wang J, Meijer J, et al. Salivary proteomic and genomic biomarkers for primary Sjogren's syndrome. Arthritis Rheum 2007;56:3588–600.
4. WM E. Saliva: its secretion, composition and functions. Braz Dent J 1992;172: 305–12.
5. Malamud D. Saliva as a diagnostic fluid. Dent Clin North Am 2011;55:159–78.
6. Park NJ, Li Y, Yu T, et al. Characterization of RNA in saliva. Clin Chem 2006;52: 988–94.
7. Park NJ, Zhou H, Elashoff D, et al. Salivary microRNA: discovery, characterization, and clinical utility for oral cancer detection. Clin Cancer Res 2009;15: 5473–7.
8. Hu S, Loo JA, Wong DT. Human saliva proteome analysis. Ann N Y Acad Sci 2007;1098:323–9.
9. Dewhirst FE, Chen T, Izard J, et al. The human oral microbiome. J Bacteriol 2010; 192:5002–17.
10. Denny P, Hagen FK, Hardt M, et al. The proteomes of human parotid and submandibular/sublingual gland salivas collected as the ductal secretions. J Proteome Res 2008;7:1994–2006.
11. Loo JA, Yan W, Ramachandran P, et al. Comparative human salivary and plasma proteomes. J Dent Res 2010;89:1016–23.
12. Yan W, Apweiler R, Balgley BM, et al. Systematic comparison of the human saliva and plasma proteomes. Proteomics Clin Appl 2009;3:116–34.
13. Mandel ID. The role of saliva in maintaining oral homeostasis. J Am Dent Assoc 1989;119:298–304.
14. Amerongen AV, Veerman EC. Saliva–the defender of the oral cavity. Oral Dis 2002;8:12–22.
15. Kaufman E, Lamster IB. The diagnostic applications of saliva–a review. Crit Rev Oral Biol Med 2002;13:197–212.
16. Burbelo PD, Bayat A, Lebovitz EE, et al. New technologies for studying the complexity of oral diseases. Oral Dis 2012;18:121–6.

17. Ruhl S. The scientific exploration of saliva in the post-proteomic era: from database back to basic function. Expert Rev Proteomics 2012;9:85–96.
18. Henson BS, Wong DT. Collection, storage, and processing of saliva samples for downstream molecular applications. Methods Mol Biol 2010;666:21–30.
19. Vitali C, Bombardieri S, Jonsson R, et al. Classification criteria for Sjogren's syndrome: a revised version of the European criteria proposed by the American-European Consensus Group. Ann Rheum Dis 2002;61:554–8.
20. Ching KH, Burbelo PD, Gonzalez-Begne M, et al. Salivary anti-Ro60 and anti-Ro52 antibody profiles to diagnose Sjogren's Syndrome. J Dent Res 2011;90: 445–9.
21. Markusse HM, Otten HG, Vroom TM, et al. Rheumatoid factor isotypes in serum and salivary fluid of patients with primary Sjogren's syndrome. Clin Immunol Immunopathol 1993;66:26–32.
22. Hu S, Vissink A, Arellano M, et al. Identification of autoantibody biomarkers for primary Sjogren's syndrome using protein microarrays. Proteomics 2011;11: 1499–507.
23. Ben-Chetrit E, Fischel R, Rubinow A. Anti-SSA/Ro and anti-SSB/La antibodies in serum and saliva of patients with Sjogren's syndrome. Clin Rheumatol 1993;12: 471–4.
24. Dunne JV, Carson DA, Spiegelberg HL, et al. IgA rheumatoid factor in the sera and saliva of patients with rheumatoid arthritis and Sjogren's syndrome. Ann Rheum Dis 1979;38:161–5.
25. Berra A, Sterin-Borda L, Bacman S, et al. Role of salivary IgA in the pathogenesis of Sjogren syndrome. Clin Immunol 2002;104:49–57.
26. Moody M, Zipp M, Al-Hashimi I. Salivary anti-spectrin autoantibodies in Sjogren's syndrome. Oral Surg Oral Med Oral Pathol Oral Radiol Endod 2001;91:322–7.
27. He J, Qiang L, Ding Y, et al. The role of muscarinic acetylcholine receptor type 3 polypeptide (M3RP205-220) antibody in the saliva of patients with primary Sjogren's syndrome. Clin Exp Rheumatol 2012;30:322–6.
28. Kang EH, Lee YJ, Hyon JY, et al. Salivary cytokine profiles in primary Sjogren's syndrome differ from those in non-Sjogren sicca in terms of TNF-alpha levels and Th-1/Th-2 ratios. Clin Exp Rheumatol 2011;29:970–6.
29. Ohyama K, Moriyama M, Hayashida JN, et al. Saliva as a potential tool for diagnosis of dry mouth including Sjogren's syndrome. Oral Dis 2015;21:224–31.
30. Rhodus N, Dahmer L, Lindemann K, et al. s-IgA and cytokine levels in whole saliva of Sjogren's syndrome patients before and after oral pilocarpine hydrochloride administration: a pilot study. Clin Oral Investig 1998;2:191–6.
31. Streckfus C, Bigler L, Navazesh M, et al. Cytokine concentrations in stimulated whole saliva among patients with primary Sjogren's syndrome, secondary Sjogren's syndrome, and patients with primary Sjogren's syndrome receiving varying doses of interferon for symptomatic treatment of the condition: a preliminary study. Clin Oral Investig 2001;5:133–5.
32. Al Kawas S, Rahim ZH, Ferguson DB. Potential uses of human salivary protein and peptide analysis in the diagnosis of disease. Arch Oral Biol 2012;57:1–9.
33. Baldini C, Giusti L, Ciregia F, et al. Proteomic analysis of saliva: a unique tool to distinguish primary Sjogren's syndrome from secondary Sjogren's syndrome and other sicca syndromes. Arthritis Res Ther 2011;13:R194.
34. Fleissig Y, Deutsch O, Reichenberg E, et al. Different proteomic protein patterns in saliva of Sjogren's syndrome patients. Oral Dis 2009;15:61–8.
35. Hu S, Gao K, Pollard R, et al. Preclinical validation of salivary biomarkers for primary Sjogren's syndrome. Arthritis Care Res 2010;62:1633–8.

36. Peluso G, De Santis M, Inzitari R, et al. Proteomic study of salivary peptides and proteins in patients with Sjogren's syndrome before and after pilocarpine treatment. Arthritis Rheum 2007;56:2216–22.
37. Ryu OH, Atkinson JC, Hoehn GT, et al. Identification of parotid salivary biomarkers in Sjogren's syndrome by surface-enhanced laser desorption/ionization time-of-flight mass spectrometry and two-dimensional difference gel electrophoresis. Rheumatology 2006;45:1077–86.
38. Ito K, Funayama S, Hitomi Y, et al. Proteome analysis of gelatin-bound salivary proteins in patients with primary Sjogren's syndrome: identification of matrix metalloproteinase-9. Clin Chim Acta 2009;403:269–71.
39. Deutsch O, Krief G, Konttinen YT, et al. Identification of Sjogren's syndrome oral fluid biomarker candidates following high-abundance protein depletion. Rheumatology 2015;54:884–90.
40. Delaleu N, Mydel P, Kwee I, et al. High fidelity between saliva proteomics and the biologic state of salivary glands defines biomarker signatures for primary Sjogren's syndrome. Arthritis Rheum 2015;67:1084–95.
41. Voulgarelis M, Skopouli FN. Clinical, immunologic, and molecular factors predicting lymphoma development in Sjogren's syndrome patients. Clin Rev Allergy Immunol 2007;32:265–74.
42. Baldini C, Pepe P, Luciano N, et al. A clinical prediction rule for lymphoma development in primary Sjogren's syndrome. J Rheumatol 2012;39:804–8.
43. Hu S, Zhou M, Jiang J, et al. Systems biology analysis of Sjogren's syndrome and mucosa-associated lymphoid tissue lymphoma in parotid glands. Arthritis Rheum 2009;60:81–92.
44. Baldini C, Giusti L, Ciregia F, et al. Correspondence between salivary proteomic pattern and clinical course in primary Sjogren syndrome and non-Hodgkin's lymphoma: a case report. J Transl Med 2011;9:188.

Polyautoimmunity in Sjögren Syndrome

Juan-Manuel Anaya, MD, PhD[a],*, Adriana Rojas-Villarraga, MD[a],
Ruben D. Mantilla, MD[a], Mauricio Arcos-Burgos, MD, PhD[b],
Juan Camilo Sarmiento-Monroy, MD[a]

KEYWORDS

- Sjögren syndrome • Polyautoimmunity • Autoimmune tautology

KEY POINTS

- Polyautoimmunity corresponds to the presence of more than one well-defined autoimmune disease in a single patient.
- Sjögren syndrome has been described in association with a large variety of both organ-specific and systemic autoimmune diseases.
- The most frequent polyautoimmunity in Sjögren syndrome is autoimmune thyroid disease.
- Main factors associated with polyautoimmunity are tobacco smoking and some genetic variants.
- The study of polyautoimmunity provides important clues for elucidating the common mechanisms of autoimmune diseases (ie, the autoimmune tautology).

INTRODUCTION

Autoimmune diseases (ADs) are chronic conditions initiated by the loss of immunologic tolerance to self-antigens due to the interaction of hereditary (ie, genetics and epigenetics) and environmental factors over time.[1] Sjögren syndrome (SS) is an AD characterized by a progressive lymphocytic and plasma cell infiltration of the salivary and lachrymal glands. It is accompanied by the production of autoantibodies leading to xerostomia and keratoconjunctivitis sicca (sicca symptoms).[2] The spectrum of the disease extends from an organ-specific autoimmune disorder (autoimmune exocrinopathy) to a systemic process involving the musculoskeletal, pulmonary, gastrointestinal,

Funding: This work was supported by the School of Medicine and Health Sciences (ABN-011), Universidad del Rosario, Bogotá, Colombia.
Conflict of Interest: No disclosures.
[a] Center for Autoimmune Diseases Research (CREA), School of Medicine and Health Sciences, Universidad del Rosario, Carrera 26 No. 63B-51, Bogotá 111221, Colombia; [b] Genomics and Predictive Medicine, Genome Biology Department, John Curtin School of Medical Research, ANU College of Medicine, Biology and Environment, The Australian National University, ACT, Garrand Road, Canberra 2600, Australia
* Corresponding author.
E-mail address: anayajm@gmail.com

hematologic, vascular, dermatologic, renal, and nervous systems (**Fig. 1**). Because the target tissue involved in the autoimmune histopathologic lesions of SS is the epithelium, the term "autoimmune epithelitis" is currently used to describe the disorder.[3]

The diagnosis of SS is based on the combination of symptoms and the presence of the autoimmune characteristics: activation of T cells (ie, positive salivary gland biopsy) or B cells (ie, presence of autoantibodies). However, not all the individuals presenting sicca symptoms have SS. The main differential diagnosis of this disorder includes the use of medications with anticholinergic effects and endocrine diseases (eg, hypothyroidism, diabetes, and hypoandrogenism). No single test of oral or ocular involvement is sufficiently sensitive and specific to form a standard diagnosis of SS. Only the simultaneous positivity of various tests with the presence of subjective symptoms and serologic abnormalities (eg, anti-Ro and anti-La antibodies) and the presence of a score that is more than a "focus score" on the minor salivary gland biopsy (ie, at least 50 cells present in 4 mm^2 of gland surface unit) allow sufficient accuracy to diagnose this condition. The classification criteria for SS are those of the American-European Consensus Group (AECG), which require either salivary gland abnormality showing

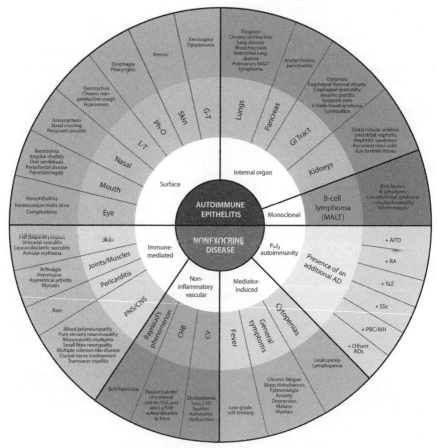

Fig. 1. Clinical spectrum of SS. AT, atherosclerosis; CHB, congenital heart block; CNS, central nervous system; CV, cardiovascular; CVD, cardiovascular disease; GI, gastrointestinal; GMN, glomerulonephritis; G-T, genital tract; L-T, laryngotracheal; MALT, mucosal-associated lymphoid tissue; Ph-O, pharyngo-esophageal; PNS, peripheral nervous system.

foci of lymphocytic infiltration or positive serology in the form of anti-Ro or anti-La antibodies.[4] Recently, new classification criteria have been proposed[5] and compared with the AECG criteria.[6]

There is compelling evidence showing that ADs share several physiopathologic mechanisms that are reflected in the clinical similarities they exhibit and in the multiple combination of ADs observed in a single patient and in their families (ie, the autoimmune tautology) (**Fig. 2**).[7] Polyautoimmunity and the multiple autoimmune syndrome (MAS) are terms used to describe the presence of more than one AD in the same patient. Polyautoimmunity refers to ADs co-occurring within patients, while MAS is a term used when a patient develops 3 or more ADs.[8,9]

Historical Perspective

Since the first description by Henrik Sjögren in 1933, it has been well known that most of the patients with this syndrome present with polyautoimmunity. In fact, of the 19 patients he originally described, 13 (68.4%) also had rheumatoid arthritis (RA).[10]

In the classical description of 62 patients with SS by Bloch and colleagues[11] in 1965, most of them had an additional AD, including RA, systemic sclerosis (SSc), or polymyositis. Moreover, Bloch and Bunim[12] were the first to suggest a shared immunopathologic mechanism for SS, systemic lupus erythematosus (SLE), SSc, and autoimmune thyroid disease (AITD) as well as a possible familial aggregation of these diseases in patients with SS. In 1979, Moutsopoulos and colleagues[13] clarified the distinction between primary and secondary SS and recommended that the disease be termed primary when it occurs alone and secondary when it is associated with another AD. Since then, the term secondary SS has been used to describe the coexistence of SS with mainly RA or SLE. However, and as is shown herein, SS may coexist with all the systemic ADs and with most of the organ-specific ADs. In this case, the authors have proposed the term polyautoimmunity,[14] which groups all the taxonomy terms referring to coexistence of well-defined ADs in a single individual because some of the terms previously used are confusing and exclude various associations. This view has been also adopted by an expert consensus, which stated that regardless of any concurrent organ-specific or multiorgan AD, SS should be diagnosed for all who fulfill the criteria they proposed without distinguishing between primary or secondary.[5]

Polyautoimmunity or Overlap Syndrome?

Polyautoimmunity was used by Sheenan and Stanton-King[15] for the first time while describing a patient with idiopathic thrombocytopenic purpura (ITP), pernicious anemia (PA), AITD, SSc, pancreatic exocrine insufficiency, and celiac disease before dying of vasculitic complications. The case they depicted corresponds to a typical MAS, which is already included in the term polyautoimmunity.

Polyautoimmunity has been referred to as overlap syndrome; some of these are frequent enough to have been given names like rhupus and sclerodermatomyositis.[14] The main difference between polyautoimmunity and the overlapping syndromes lies in the fact that the former is the presence of 2 or more well-defined autoimmune conditions fulfilling validated classification criteria, whereas the latter is the partial presence of signs and symptoms of diverse ADs. Most of the cases of overlapping syndromes have been described in cross-sectional studies. As has been shown, there is a lag in the time interval between the first and the second AD.[16] For example, in the mixed connective tissue disease (MCTD), the classical overlap syndrome, some patients will develop SLE, SSc, or RA during the course of the disease, and some will present with a longstanding MCTD.[17] Long-term studies have shown that MCTD remains an

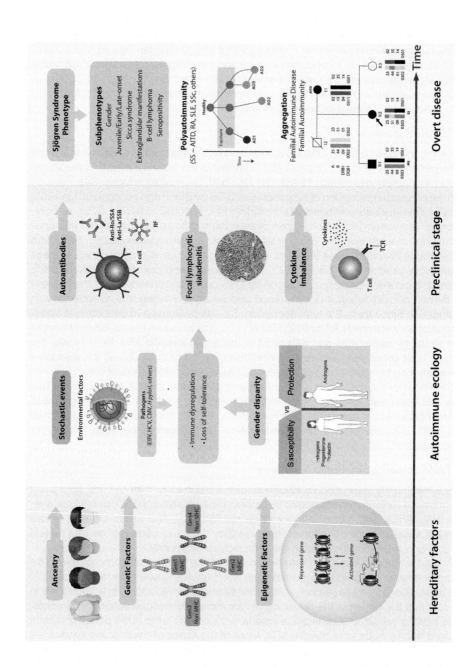

overlap syndrome in about 60% of the patients. The remaining 40% progress to SSc, SLE, or RA,[18] highlighting the fact that ADs are a spectrum ranging from the incomplete forms or "forme frustre" and lenient and slow evolution syndromes to the rapidly progressive and fatal forms (see **Fig. 1**). The imbalance between permissive and protective factors (ie, hereditary and environmental) interacting over time may explain this spectrum[1] and the fact that "there are no diseases but rather patients."

POLYAUTOIMMUNITY IN SJÖGREN SYNDROME

SS has been described in association with a large variety of ADs including AITD, RA, SLE, SSc, autoimmune hepatitis (AIH), and primary biliary cirrhosis (PBC), and the like[19–21] (**Table 1**). Lockshin and colleagues[22] reported a prevalence of polyautoimmunity in 52% of their patients with SS (defined by ophthalmologist-prescribed artificial tears or punctal plugs, salivary gland hypertrophy, and/or cryoglobulinemia). Patients with polyautoimmunity differed from those with "pure" SS regarding race (ie, "non-white").

Amador-Patarroyo and colleagues[21] assessed a cohort of 410 patients with SS and observed a prevalence of polyautoimmunity in 32.6% of them. The most frequent and closely coexistent diseases were AITD (21.5%), RA (8.3%), SLE (7.6%), and inflammatory bowel disease (0.7%), which together constituted a cluster group. There were 35 (8.5%) patients with MAS. Similar results were reported by Lazarus and Isenberg.[23] As a corollary, patients with SS should be monitored on a regular basis for polyautoimmunity.

Sjögren Syndrome and Autoimmune Hepatitis

Endocrine symptoms documented in SS patients are mainly due to concomitant thyroid dysfunction.[24] Between 15% and 30% of patients with SS develop AITD, primarily Hashimoto thyroiditis (HT).[25] Patients with SS seropositive for antithyroid peroxidase and antithyroglobulin antibodies are at risk of future thyroid disease.[25]

The prevalence of SS is 10 times higher in patients with autoimmune thyroiditis.[26] It is advisable that patients with SS be screened periodically for thyroid function.[26] The association of HT in patients suffering from SS defines a subset of patients with milder disease and normal C4 levels.[27] The histologic picture of HT per se is highly similar to that of SS.[28] HT may evolve to lymphoma in 0.5% of patients.[29] One-third of the patients with AITD have SS features, and one of 10 antinuclear antibody (ANA) -positive AITD patients shares the diagnosis of SS.[28]

Fig. 2. Fourth-stage model for the pathophysiology of ADs (eg, SS). Each stage shows the known phenomena that, when it has accumulated, will be the causative scenario for the onset of ADs. First, heritable factors have an impact over the life of the individuals. They converge and interact to increase or decrease the risk an individual would have of developing the disease. Second, the autoimmune ecology corresponds to the effect of environmental factors, which, acting stochastically, will also influence the risk and course of disease. Once the autoimmune tolerance is lost by the interaction of heritable and environmental factors, a preclinical stage characterized by B- and T-cell dysregulation arises. This third phase may take years before the phenotype becomes clinically evident. The clinical stage has a broad spectrum of subphenotypes that can influence outcomes, treatment, and mortality. Note that familial autoimmunity corresponds to the presence of different ADs in a nuclear family. AOD, age at onset of disease; CMV, cytomegalovirus; EBV, Epstein-Barr virus; HCV, hepatitis C virus; MHC, major histocompatibility complex; RF, rheumatoid factor; TCR, T-cell receptor.

Table 1
Sjögren syndrome and polyautoimmunity

Variable	SS	Phenotype			
		SS			
		+AITD	+RA	+SLE	+SSc
Prevalence	0.1%–4.8%	15%–30%	4%–31%	9%–19%	14%
Autoimmune profile	Anti-Ro/SSA (33%–74%) Anti-La/SSB (23%–52%) RF (36%–74%) ACPA (3%–10%) ANA (59%–85%)[a]	Anti-TPO Anti-Tg ANA	ACPA (71.4%) Anti-Ro/SSA and anti-La/SSB (12%)	Higher RF, anti-Ro/SSA, and anti-La/SSB Anti-La/SSB as serologic marker	ACA (37%) Anti-SCL70 (13%) Anti-Ro/SSA (39%) Anti-La/SSB (22%) Anti-RNA Pol (2%)
Physiopathology	Focal lymphocytic sialadenitis (minor salivary glands), with a focus score ≥1 SS may be associated with organ damage due to several mechanisms	Infiltrate consists of primarily CD4+ T lymphocytes The thyroid epithelial cells express HLA class II molecules and adhesion molecules	Differences in genetic and immunologic pathways	Sharing many immunogenetic features	Lymphocytic infiltration of salivary glands leading to oral dryness is one of the main features in SS as well as salivary gland fibrosis

Subphenotype characteristics	SS has a wide clinical spectrum that extends from benign local exocrinopathy to systemic disorder that affects several organs	Milder disease and normal C4 levels	Articular involvement and RA activity are independent of SS	Milder SLE-related features and a predominance of SS-related features	Limited SSc predominantly associated
Prognosis	Lymphoma (5%–10%)	Progress to B-cell MALT lymphoma is probable Lymphoma (0.5%)	Doubled standardized incidence ratio for NHL	Lower risk of developing glomerulonephritis	SS may be protective against SSc-associated pulmonary fibrosis
Treatment approach	Immunosuppressant agents (eg, CsA, AZA, MTX, MMF, and LEF are all used empirically in SS with extraglandular manifestations)	No immunosuppressant agents required	Corticosteroids and immunosuppressants (eg, methotrexate) Rituximab may be considered in refractory cases	HCQS, corticosteroids, and in more severe cases immunosuppressants have been effectively used, including Rituximab	In refractory or severe cases, immunosuppressants, such as AZA, MMF, or CYC, have to be considered High-dose IVIg can be an effective option

Abbreviations: ACA, anticentromere antibodies; anti-Tg, antithyroglobulin antibodies; anti-TPO, antithyroid peroxidase antibodies; AZA, azathioprine; CsA, cyclosporine A; CYC, cyclophosphamide; HCQS, hydroxychloroquine; IVIg, intravenous immunoglobulin; LEF, leflunomide; MALT, mucosal-associated lymphoid tissue; MMF, mycophenolate mofetil; MTX, methotrexate; RF, rheumatoid factor; SSA, Anti SS related antigen A antibodies (Ro/SSA antibodies); SSB, Anti-SS related antigen B antibodies (La/SSB antibodies); TNF, tumor necrosis factor.

[a] Other autoantibodies described in SS patients: ACA (3.7%–27%), anti-SCL70 (<5%), AMA (1.7%–13%), and ASMA (30%–62%).

[b] Mainly HT. Prevalence of SS corresponds to the general population. Prevalence of AITD, RA, SLE, and SSc corresponds to that observed associated with SS.

Adapted from Iaccarino L, Gatto M, Bettio S, et al. Overlap connective tissue disease syndromes. Autoimmun Rev 2013;12(3):363–73.

Sjögren Syndrome and Rheumatoid Arthritis

RA is frequently associated with both sicca symptoms and true SS. Patients with RA may show evidence of dry eye regardless of the coexistence of SS or other concomitant disease.[30] The prevalence of sicca symptoms in patients with RA ranges from 30% to 50%,[31,32] and the percentage of RA patients who fulfill SS classification criteria ranges from 4% to 31%.[31–33] Arthralgia arthritis, in turn, is reported in 70% of SS patients. Many investigators consider SS an extra-articular manifestation of RA, although differences in genetic and immunologic pathways involved in the disease process have been documented.[31]

Prevalence of anticitrullinated protein antibodies (ACPA) has been reported in 7.2% of patients with SS who are RF negative and without arthritis.[34] Median-term follow-up of ACPA-positive patients with SS showed that almost half of them developed RA, particularly in the presence of elevated acute phase reactants.[35] In the authors' series, ACPA were observed in 9% of SS patients, of whom 80% were RF positive.[36] This prevalence was higher (67%) in SS-RA patients.[36] Iwamoto and colleagues[37] detected ACPA in 21% of SS patients with arthritis and in none of those without arthritis. Notably, ACPA were found in 71.4% of patients classified as having SS-RA and in 6% of SS patients with arthritis but without RA. RF is not helpful for differentiating patients with SS from those with SS-RA polyautoimmunity. SS-RA patients are less frequently anti-Ro and anti-La antibody positive than patients with SS (12% vs 82%).[38]

The number of joints involved and the activity of RA are independent of the presence of SS.[39] A 17% cumulative prevalence of SS was described in a Spanish cohort of RA patients.[40] Similar results were observed in an Austrian cohort.[41] In Finland, a doubling of the standardized incidence ratio for non-Hodgkin lymphoma (NHL) in RA patients with polyautoimmunity when compared with RA patients without SS was described.[42]

Sjögren Syndrome and Systemic Lupus Erythematosus

SLE is probably the AD most closely related to SS due to the significant overlap in their clinical and immunologic expression. The prevalence of sicca syndrome in SLE ranges between 18% and 34%.[20] Recent studies have described a prevalence of associated SS in SLE patients ranging between 9% and 19%.[31,43,44] In a large prospective series, skin involvement, such as photosensitivity or malar rash, oral ulcers, arthritis, Raynaud phenomenon, and psychosis, were reported more frequently in the SS-SLE group.[45] SS-SLE patients are older with a lower risk of developing glomerulonephritis compared with SLE patients.[45] Other investigators reported a higher frequency of fatigue and thrombocytopenia in SS-SLE patients.[43] A meta-analysis disclosed a 17.8% prevalence of SS.[46] SS-SLE patients constitute a subphenotype characterized by milder SLE-related features and a predominance of SS-related features.[31,43] One study found patients with SS-SLE were also more likely to have AITD compared with those with only SLE.[47] In summary, the polyautoimmunity SS-SLE seems to be characterized by less organ involvement, a more specific autoantibody profile, and a favorable clinical outcome.

Among families identified by the presence of SLE, both "primary" and "secondary" SS tend to occur within the same families.[48] Aggarwal and colleagues mentioned in their article "These results highlight the commonalities between these two forms of SS, which in fact correspond to the same disease."[48]

Sjögren Syndrome and Systemic Sclerosis

Sicca symptoms are common in SSc because they are observed in 68% to 83% of the cases. However, only 14% of SSc-sicca patients fulfill the criteria for SS.[49] SS-SSc is more often complicated by peripheral neuropathy and additional ADs or autoantibodies not typical for either SS or SSc alone.[19,49]

Digital ulcers were reported in 11.8% of the cases and pulmonary hypertension in 23.6%. In SS-SSc, skin involvement seems to be less severe than in SSc patients and the incidence of digital ulcers lower.[50] SS may be protective against SSc-associated pulmonary fibrosis. Limited SSc was predominantly associated with SS in these studies.[47]

Sjögren Syndrome and Hepatic Autoimmune Diseases

Liver involvement was one of the first systemic manifestations reported in SS.[51] After eliminating hepatotoxic drugs and fatty liver disease, the 2 main causes of liver disease in SS are chronic viral infections and autoimmune liver diseases, which require different therapeutic approaches and have different prognoses.[52] With respect to viral infections, chronic HCV infection is the main cause of liver involvement in SS patients from the Mediterranean area, whereas chronic HBV infection may be the main cause of liver involvement in SS patients from Asian countries.[52]

After eliminating viral hepatitis, PBC should be considered the main cause of liver disease in SS.[52] PBC-SS patients may have a broad spectrum of abnormalities of the liver. In fact, the comparison of liver histology between the PBC with SS patient group and the PBC without SS patient group showed that the incidence of lymphoid nonsuppurative cholangitis was higher in PBC-SS patients.[53] SS has been shown to be the most common AD complicating concomitant SLE and PBC.[54] Serologically, the diagnostic hallmark of PBC is the presence of significant titers of antimitochondrial antibodies (AMA), which is possibly the most specific autoantibody in clinical immunology.[52]

AIH is diagnosed in 1.7% to 4% of patients with SS.[55] AIH is the second most frequently observed autoimmune liver disease in SS (all reported cases are type I), and nearly 10% of these patients may have AIH-PBC.[56] Only 10% of SS-related type I AIH patients may have positive AMA (AIH-PBC); therefore, AMA could discriminate between PBC and AIH.[52] In an evaluation of polyautoimmunity in AIH, SS was the most frequent (15.2%).[57] When the prevalence of concurrent extrahepatic AD in patients with AIH/PBC polyautoimmunity was assessed, SS was observed in 8.4%, which corresponds to the MAS phenotype.[58]

SEVERITY OF POLYAUTOIMMUNITY

Polyautoimmunity may impact the outcome of ADs. In the case of SS-SLE and SS-SSc patients, several investigators suggest a more benign course of SLE and SSc, respectively, and therefore, a better prognosis.

SS-SLE patients have a lower risk of developing glomerulonephritis compared with SLE patients. The coexistence of SS in patients with SLE does not affect the severity of SLE.[59] Rather, it seems to be a protective factor against the development of lupus nephritis.[43,45] In terms of treatment, the efficacy and safety of rituximab therapy in patients with refractory ITP and SLE and/or SS were evaluated. All patients with SS had a complete response to treatment.[60]

Patients with NHL associated with SLE had sicca symptoms, salivary gland swelling, and anti-Ro and anti-La antibodies significantly more often than patients with SLE alone.[61] SS disease severity has been shown to be the strongest predictor of swallowing disorders, but these disorders did not differ on the basis of SS polyautoimmunity or SS alone.[62] A more frequent lung involvement (25% vs 8.1%; $P = .05$) has been found in patients with SS and ACPA positivity.[35]

As mentioned, skin involvement in limited SSc seems to be less severe when it appears in SSc-SS, and the incidence of digital ulcers is lower than that reported in SSc patients.[50] Furthermore, SS may be protective against SSc-associated pulmonary fibrosis.[63] The explanation for these phenomena requires further analysis in order to understand the physiopathogenic pathways underlying this apparent protective effect.

FACTORS ASSOCIATED WITH POLYAUTOIMMUNITY IN SJÖGREN SYNDROME

Besides duration of disease, both genetics and environmental factors have been reported to be associated with polyautoimmunity in SS.[21,64]

In a study in which patients with SS and polyautoimmunity were evaluated by whole exome sequencing, novel and rare mutations were identified.[64] Among them, those harbored by the *LRP1/STAT6* locus were considered the strongest causative factors for polyautoimmunity. *LRP1/STAT6* mutation is involved in extracellular and intracellular anti-inflammatory pathways that play key roles in maintaining the homeostasis of the immune system. A lack of influence of Th17 polymorphisms on the susceptibility and severity of SS-RA polyautoimmunity was recently reported.[65]

Smoking per se is considered a risk factor for both the development of ADs, such as RA, SLE, and AITD, and the positivity of autoantibodies.[66] Pathophysiologic mechanisms have been described including influence on lymphocytic and plasma cell functions, apoptosis and effects on cytokines, and hormonal imbalances. A controversial effect of habitual smoking on the spectrum of the disease has been reported in SS. Manthorpe and colleagues[67] showed that SS patients who smoked had anti-Ro and anti-La antibodies less frequently and a lower focus score than those who did not smoke. They explain that smoking may lower the focus score by reducing the lymphocyte infiltration in salivary glands, thus reducing the production of anti-Ro and anti-La antibodies. Karabulut and colleagues[68] showed an association between SS, ANA titers, and habitual smoking. In addition, positive smoking status was associated with polyautoimmunity in SS patients.[21]

The association between polyautoimmunity and low socioeconomic status in SS patients has been highlighted.[69] This finding is in concordance with the influence of socioeconomic status on chronic diseases in which low socioeconomic status is associated with morbidity and mortality.[70]

The influence of infection on polyautoimmunity has been evaluated in some studies. Vasculitis in SS patients was associated with the presence of immunoglobulin G *Saccharomyces cerevisiae* antibodies.[71] These results may be related to the fact that microbe-activating specific innate immune responses are critical, whereas antigenic cross-reactivity may perpetuate immune responses leading to chronic autoinflammatory disease.[72] There are numerous case reports or case series showing the association with an infectious agent (varicella zoster, Epstein-Barr virus, *Helicobacter pylori* infection, hepatitis C virus) and polyautoimmunity in SS.[73]

AUTOIMMUNE TAUTOLOGY AND SJÖGREN SYNDROME

Polyautoimmunity is one of the major arguments supporting the autoimmune tautology (ie, the common mechanisms of ADs) due to the fact that in an individual with 2 or more diseases, the same genetic background, and the same environment influence the appearance of different phenotypes. Ten characteristics supporting this logically valid propositional theory applied to SS are shown in **Table 2**.

Table 2
Sjögren syndrome in light of the autoimmune tautology

Characteristic	Description
Female preponderance	Female-to-male ratio as high as 10:1. Some studies have found differences with respect to immunologic, clinical, and severity features (including lymphoma risk) in men with SS.
Shared subphenotypes	Sicca symptoms are nonspecific. Another AD (eg, RA, SSc) could manifest with dry mouth and eyes. Several systemic manifestations of SS are present in other autoimmune conditions. Autoantibodies (ie, ANA, anti-Ro, anti-La, rheumatoid factor) are not specific to SS and may be present in other ADs.
Polyautoimmunity	SS has been described in association with a large variety of ADs, both organ-specific (eg, AITD, multiple sclerosis, PBC, AIH) and systemic (eg, RA, SLE, SSc).
Familial autoimmunity	Familial coaggregation of ADs has been reported in up to 38% of patients with SS with AITD, SLE, and RA being the most frequent.
Similar pathophysiology	Damage induced by T or B cells, or both, plays a major pathogenic role in ADs. Although the autoimmune phenotype varies depending on the target cell and the affected organ, the local mechanisms for tissue injury are similar (eg, activation of the type I interferon pathway, decreased T- and B-regulatory functions). Focal lymphocytic aggregates are the histopathologic hallmark of SS, but they are similar to the inflammatory infiltrate seen in organ-specific ADs (eg, type 1 diabetes, AITD).
Autoimmune ecology	Environmental factors, including infectious agents (eg, EBV, CMV), vitamin D deficiency, and smoking are associated with SS and other ADs.
Influence of age of onset	Although SS is a late-onset disease, clinical manifestations of juvenile SS may vary more than those seen in adult patients (eg, lower frequency of sicca syndrome, higher rates of parotid enlargement, higher prevalence of immunologic markers).
Influence of ancestry	The highest rates of SS are documented in northern Europe, while the rates in North America and mainland Europe seem to be comparable, and the lowest rates are observed in some parts of Asia. Note that nothing is published on detailed series of SS cases in African descendents.
Common genetic factors	The genetic risk factors for ADs consist of 2 forms, those common to many conditions and those specific to a given disorder. SS shares genetic factors at the MHC and non-MHC loci with several other ADs.
Similar treatment	In addition to sicca treatment, patients with SS (mainly those with systemic manifestations) may benefit from immunosuppressive treatment (eg, corticosteroids, cyclophosphamide, methotrexate) and antimalarials. In refractory cases, B-cell depletion therapy may be considered.

Abbreviations: CMV, cytomegalovirus; EBV, Epstein-Barr virus; MHC, major histocompatibility complex.

FUTURE CONSIDERATIONS

Based on polyautoimmunity and depending on severity, ADs may be categorized as major and minor conditions. In this sense, how polyautoimmunity affects major ADs warrants further investigation. In turn, the identification of commonalities among ADs may provide insights about salient mechanisms that are necessary and perhaps sufficient for autoimmunity to occur (see **Fig. 2**). Last, polyautoimmunity, as an extreme phenotype of autoimmunity, would be critical for dissecting genes of major effect conferring susceptibility to autoimmunity. Assessment and clustering of polyautoimmunity in SS and other ADs will help to define plausible approaches to studying the autoimmune tautology.

SUMMARY

Polyautoimmunity is a frequent condition in SS and follows a grouping pattern. The most frequent ADs observed in SS are AITD, RA, and SLE. Genetic and environmental factors influence the development of polyautoimmunity.

REFERENCES

1. Anaya J-M, Rojas-Villarraga A, Schoenfeld Y. From de mosaic of autoimmunity to the autoimmune tautology. In: Anaya J-M, Schoenfeld Y, Rojas-Villarraga A, et al, editors. Autoimmunity from bench to bedside. First. Bogotá (Colombia): El Rosario University Press; 2013. p. 237–45.
2. Anaya JM, Talal N. Sjögren's syndrome comes of age. Semin Arthritis Rheum 1999;28(6):355–9.
3. Moutsopoulos HM. Sjögren's syndrome: autoimmune epithelitis. Clin Immunol Immunopathol 1994;72(2):162–5.
4. Vitali C, Bombardieri S, Jonsson R, et al. Classification criteria for Sjögren's syndrome: a revised version of the European criteria proposed by the American-European Consensus Group. Ann Rheum Dis 2002;61(6):554–8.
5. Shiboski SC, Shiboski CH, Criswell LA, et al. American College of Rheumatology classification criteria for Sjögren's syndrome: a data-driven, expert consensus approach in the Sjögren's International Collaborative Clinical Alliance cohort. Arthritis Care Res (Hoboken) 2012;64(4):475–87.
6. Rasmussen A, Ice JA, Li H, et al. Comparison of the American-European Consensus Group Sjogren's syndrome classification criteria to newly proposed American College of Rheumatology criteria in a large, carefully characterised sicca cohort. Ann Rheum Dis 2014;73(1):31–8.
7. Anaya J-M. The autoimmune tautology. Arthritis Res Ther 2010;12(6):147.
8. Anaya J M, Corena R. Castiblanco J, et al. The kaleidoscope of autoimmunity: multiple autoimmune syndromes and familial autoimmunity. Expert Rev Clin Immunol 2007;3(4):623–35.
9. Anaya J-M. The diagnosis and clinical significance of polyautoimmunity. Autoimmun Rev 2014;13(4–5):423–6.
10. Sjögren H. Zur Kenntnis der Keratoconjunctivitis (Keratitis Filiformis bei Hypofunktion der Tränendrüsen). Acta Ophthalmol 1933;11:1–151.
11. Bloch KJ, Buchanan WW, Wohl MJ, et al. Sjögren's syndrome. A clinical, pathological, and serological study of sixty-two cases. Medicine (Baltimore) 1965;44: 187–231.
12. Bloch KJ, Bunim JJ. Sjögren's syndrome and its relation to connective tissue diseases. J Chronic Dis 1963;16:915–27.
13. Moutsopoulos HM, Webber BL, Vlagopoulos TP, et al. Differences in the clinical manifestations of sicca syndrome in the presence and absence of rheumatoid arthritis. Am J Med 1979;66(5):733–6.
14. Rojas-Villarraga A, Amaya-Amaya J, Rodriguez-Rodriguez A, et al. Introducing polyautoimmunity: secondary autoimmune diseases no longer exist. Autoimmune Dis 2012;2012(1):254319.

15. Sheehan NJ, Stanton-King K. Polyautoimmunity in a young woman. Br J Rheumatol 1993;32(3):254–6.
16. Anaya J-M, Castiblanco J, Rojas-Villarraga A, et al. The multiple autoimmune syndromes. A clue for the autoimmune tautology. Clin Rev Allergy Immunol 2012; 43(3):256–64.
17. Venables PJW. Mixed connective tissue disease. Lupus 2006;15(3):132–7.
18. Cappelli S, Bellando Randone S, Martinović D, et al. "To be or not to be," ten years after: evidence for mixed connective tissue disease as a distinct entity. Semin Arthritis Rheum 2012;41(4):589–98.
19. Salliot C, Gottenberg J, Bengoufa D, et al. Anticentromere antibodies identify patients with Sjögren's syndrome and autoimmune overlap syndrome. J Rheumatol 2007;34(11):2253–8.
20. Iaccarino L, Gatto M, Bettio S, et al. Overlap connective tissue disease syndromes. Autoimmun Rev 2013;12(3):363–73.
21. Amador-Patarroyo MJ, Arbelaez JG, Mantilla RD, et al. Sjögren's syndrome at the crossroad of polyautoimmunity. J Autoimmun 2012;39(3):199–205.
22. Lockshin MD, Levine AB, Erkan D. Patients with overlap autoimmune disease differ from those with "pure" disease. Lupus Sci Med 2015;2(1):e000084.
23. Lazarus MN, Isenberg DA. Development of additional autoimmune diseases in a population of patients with primary Sjögren's syndrome. Ann Rheum Dis 2005; 64(7):1062–4.
24. Sarmiento-Monroy J, Mantilla R, Rojas-Villarraga A, et al. Sjögren's syndrome. In: Anaya J, Shoenfeld Y, Rojas-Villarraga A, et al, editors. Autoimmunity from bench to bedside. Bogotá (Colombia): El Rosario University Press; 2013. p. 475–517.
25. Mavragani CP, Fragoulis GE, Moutsopoulos HM. Endocrine alterations in primary Sjogren's syndrome: an overview. J Autoimmun 2012;39(4):354–8.
26. Al-Hashimi I, Khuder S, Haghighat N, et al. Frequency and predictive value of the clinical manifestations in Sjögren's syndrome. J Oral Pathol Med 2001;30(1):1–6.
27. Caramaschi P, Biasi D, Caimmi C, et al. The co-occurrence of Hashimoto thyroiditis in primary Sjogren's syndrome defines a subset of patients with milder clinical phenotype. Rheumatol Int 2013;33(5):1271–5.
28. Mitsias DI, Kapsogeorgou EK, Moutsopoulos HM. Sjögren's syndrome: why autoimmune epithelitis? Oral Dis 2006;12(6):523–32.
29. Aozasa K. Hashimoto's thyroiditis as a risk factor of thyroid lymphoma. Acta Pathol Jpn 1990;40(7):459–68.
30. Villani E, Galimberti D, Viola F, et al. Corneal involvement in rheumatoid arthritis: an in vivo confocal study. Invest Ophthalmol Vis Sci 2008;49(2):560–4.
31. Gilboe IM, Kvien TK, Uhlig T, et al. Sicca symptoms and secondary Sjögren's syndrome in systemic lupus erythematosus: comparison with rheumatoid arthritis and correlation with disease variables. Ann Rheum Dis 2001;60(12):1103–9.
32. Uhlig T, Kvien TK, Jensen JL, et al. Sicca symptoms, saliva and tear production, and disease variables in 636 patients with rheumatoid arthritis. Ann Rheum Dis 1999;58(7):415–22.
33. Mattey DL, González-Gay MA, Hajeer AH, et al. Association between HLA-DRB1*15 and secondary Sjögren's syndrome in patients with rheumatoid arthritis. J Rheumatol 2000;27(11):2611–6.
34. Gottenberg J-E, Mignot S, Nicaise-Rolland P, et al. Prevalence of anti-cyclic citrullinated peptide and anti-keratin antibodies in patients with primary Sjögren's syndrome. Ann Rheum Dis 2005;64(1):114–7.

35. Payet J, Belkhir R, Gottenberg JE, et al. ACPA-positive primary Sjögren's syndrome: true primary or rheumatoid arthritis-associated Sjögren's syndrome? RMD Open 2015;1(1):e000066.

36. Tobón GJ, Correa PA, Anaya J-M. Anti-cyclic citrullinated peptide antibodies in patients with primary Sjögren's syndrome. Ann Rheum Dis 2005;64(5):791–2.

37. Iwamoto N, Kawakami A, Tamai M, et al. Determination of the subset of Sjogren's syndrome with articular manifestations by anticyclic citrullinated peptide antibodies. J Rheumatol 2009;36(1):113–5.

38. Hernández-Molina G, Avila-Casado C, Cárdenas-Velázquez F, et al. Similarities and differences between primary and secondary Sjögren's syndrome. J Rheumatol 2010;37(4):800–8.

39. Antero DC, Parra AGM, Miyazaki FH, et al. Secondary Sjögren's syndrome and disease activity of rheumatoid arthritis. Rev Assoc Med Bras 2013;57(3):319–22.

40. Carmona L, González-Alvaro I, Balsa A, et al. Rheumatoid arthritis in Spain: occurrence of extra-articular manifestations and estimates of disease severity. Ann Rheum Dis 2003;62(9):897–900.

41. Skoumal M, Wottawa A. Long-term observation study of Austrian patients with rheumatoid arthritis. Acta Med Austriaca 2002;29(2):52–6.

42. Kauppi M, Pukkala E, Isomäki H. Elevated incidence of hematologic malignancies in patients with Sjögren's syndrome compared with patients with rheumatoid arthritis (Finland). Cancer Causes Control 1997;8(2):201–4.

43. Manoussakis MN, Georgopoulou C, Zintzaras E, et al. Sjögren's syndrome associated with systemic lupus erythematosus: clinical and laboratory profiles and comparison with primary Sjögren's syndrome. Arthritis Rheum 2004;50(3):882–91.

44. Nossent JC, Swaak AJ. Systemic lupus erythematosus VII: frequency and impact of secondary Sjøgren's syndrome. Lupus 1998;7(4):231–4.

45. Baer AN, Maynard JW, Shaikh F, et al. Secondary Sjogren's syndrome in systemic lupus erythematosus defines a distinct disease subset. J Rheumatol 2010;37(6): 1143–9.

46. Yao Q, Altman RD, Wang X. Systemic lupus erythematosus with Sjögren syndrome compared to systemic lupus erythematosus alone: a meta-analysis. J Clin Rheumatol 2012;18(1):28–32.

47. Scofield RH, Brunor GR, Harley JB, et al. Autoimmune thyroid disease is associated with a diagnosis of secondary Sjögren's syndrome in familial systemic lupus. Ann Rheum Dis 2007;66:410–3.

48. Aggarwal R, Anaya J-M, Koelsch KA, et al. Association between secondary and primary Sjögren's syndrome in a large collection of lupus families. Autoimmune Dis 2015;2015:298506.

49. Avouac J, Sordet C, Depinay C, et al. Systemic sclerosis-associated Sjögren's syndrome and relationship to the limited cutaneous subtype: results of a prospective study of sicca syndrome in 133 consecutive patients. Arthritis Rheum 2006;54(7):2243–9.

50. Hunzelmann N, Genth E, Krieg T, et al. The registry of the German Network for Systemic Scleroderma: frequency of disease subsets and patterns of organ involvement. Rheumatology (Oxford) 2008;47(8):1185–92.

51. Zeron PB, Retamozo S, Bové A, et al. Diagnosis of liver involvement in primary Sjögren syndrome. J Clin Transl Hepatol 2013;1(2):94–102.

52. Ramos-Casals M, Sánchez-Tapias J-M, Parés A, et al. Characterization and differentiation of autoimmune versus viral liver involvement in patients with Sjögren's syndrome. J Rheumatol 2006;33(8):1593–9.

53. Matsumoto T, Morizane T, Aoki Y, et al. Autoimmune hepatitis in primary Sjogren's syndrome: pathological study of the livers and labial salivary glands in 17 patients with primary Sjogren's syndrome. Pathol Int 2005;55(2):70–6.

54. Shizuma T. Clinical characteristics of concomitant systemic lupus erythematosus and primary biliary cirrhosis: a literature review. J Immunol Res 2015;2015:713728.

55. Ebert EC. Gastrointestinal and hepatic manifestations of Sjogren syndrome. J Clin Gastroenterol 2012;46(1):25–30.

56. Lindgren S, Manthorpe R, Eriksson S. Autoimmune liver disease in patients with primary Sjögren's syndrome. J Hepatol 1994;20(3):354–8.

57. Paredes Millán M, Chirinos Montes NJ, Martinez Apaza A, et al. The most common rheumatic diseases in patients with autoimmune liver disease in the Hospital Arzobispo Loayza from 2008-2013, Lima, Peru. Rev Gastroenterol Peru 2014; 34(4):305–10.

58. Efe C, Wahlin S, Ozaslan E, et al. Autoimmune hepatitis/primary biliary cirrhosis overlap syndrome and associated extrahepatic autoimmune diseases. Eur J Gastroenterol Hepatol 2012;24(5):531–4.

59. Rojas-Villarraga A, Toro C-E, Espinosa G, et al. Factors influencing polyautoimmunity in systemic lupus erythematosus. Autoimmun Rev 2010;9(4):229–32.

60. Jiang B, Li T, Guo L, et al. Efficacy and safety of rituximab in systemic lupus erythematosus and Sjögren syndrome patients with refractory thrombocytopenia. J Clin Rheumatol 2015;21(5):244–50.

61. Löfström B, Backlin C, Sundström C, et al. A closer look at non-Hodgkin's lymphoma cases in a national Swedish systemic lupus erythematosus cohort: a nested case-control study. Ann Rheum Dis 2007;66(12):1627–32.

62. Pierce JL, Tanner K, Merrill RM, et al. Swallowing disorders in Sjögren's syndrome: prevalence, risk factors, and effects on quality of life. Dysphagia 2015; 31:49–59.

63. Balbir-Gurman A, Braun-Moscovici Y. Scleroderma overlap syndrome. Isr Med Assoc J 2011;13(1):14–20.

64. Johar AS, Mastronardi C, Rojas-Villarraga A, et al. Novel and rare functional genomic variants in multiple autoimmune syndrome and Sjögren's syndrome. J Transl Med 2015;13:173.

65. Carvalho CN, do Carmo RF, Duarte ALP, et al. IL-17A and IL-17F polymorphisms in rheumatoid arthritis and Sjögren's syndrome. Clin Oral Investig 2015;20: 495–502.

66. Freemer MM, King TE, Criswell LA. Association of smoking with dsDNA autoantibody production in systemic lupus erythematosus. Ann Rheum Dis 2006;65(5): 581–4.

67. Manthorpe R, Benoni C, Jacobsson L, et al. Lower frequency of focal lip sialadenitis (focus score) in smoking patients. Can tobacco diminish the salivary gland involvement as judged by histological examination and anti-SSA/Ro and anti-SSB/La antibodies in Sjögren's syndrome? Ann Rheum Dis 2000;59(1): 54–60.

68. Karabulut G, Kitapcioglu G, Inal V, et al. Cigarette smoking in primary Sjögren's syndrome: positive association only with ANA positivity. Mod Rheumatol 2011; 21(6):602–7.

69. Anaya J-M, Amaya-Amaya J, Amador-Patarroyo MJ, et al. Influence of low socioeconomic status on autoimmune rheumatic diseases. Ann Rheum Dis 2012; 71(Suppl3):714.

70. Calixto O-J, Anaya J-M. Socioeconomic status. The relationship with health and autoimmune diseases. Autoimmun Rev 2014;13(6):641–54.

71. Kivity S, Arango MT, Ehrenfeld M, et al. Infection and autoimmunity in Sjogren's syndrome: a clinical study and comprehensive review. J Autoimmun 2014;51:17–22.

72. Root-Bernstein R, Fairweather D. Complexities in the relationship between infection and autoimmunity. Curr Allergy Asthma Rep 2014;14(1):407.

73. Jayarangaiah A, Sehgal R, Epperla N. Sjögren's syndrome and neuromyelitis optica spectrum disorders (NMOSD)–a case report and review of literature. BMC Neurol 2014;14:200.

Salivary Gland Pathology in Sjögren's Syndrome

 CrossMark

Joana Campos, PhD[a], Maarten R. Hillen, PhD[a,b], Francesca Barone, MD, PhD[a,*]

KEYWORDS

- Primary Sjögren's syndrome • Salivary glands • Histopathology
- Autoimmune disease

KEY POINTS

- The salivary glands provide the hub of primary Sjögren's syndrome (pSS) pathology.
- Several disease-defining processes have been identified that bridge the innate and acquired immune response, but how these processes interact with each other is not clear.
- The pathogenic role of local germinal center (GC) formation in lymphoma development and its relationship to LESA formation has to be established.
- Analysis of the salivary glands will hopefully provide a tool for patient stratification.

INTRODUCTION

pSS can be considered a systemic autoimmune disease with a strong organ bias. The involvement of the exocrine glands is prevalent and drives the pathognomonic manifestations of dryness that define the sicca syndrome.[1] Although the involvement of the ocular glands and the mucosal exocrine glands in the respiratory and gastrointestinal systems is less studied, the accessibility of minor and major salivary gland tissue has dramatically contributed to the understanding of pSS pathogenesis. Differently from other diseases, where target organs embody disease casualties (eg, the kidneys in lupus or the lungs in vasculitides), there is clear evidence that the salivary glands represent both the pathogenic hub of pSS and its end target. Salivary glands provide the local source of autoantigens,[2] ectopic signals for lymphocyte organization and survival,[3,4] and the microenvironment that supports autoantibody production.[5]

Disclosures: None.
[a] Centre for Translational Inflammation Research, Institute of Inflammation and Ageing, ARUK Center for the Pathogenesis of Rheumatoid Arthritis, University of Birmingham, Queen Elizabeth Hospital, Mindelsohn Way, Birmingham B15 2WB, UK; [b] Laboratory of Translational Immunology, University Medical Centre Utrecht, Heidelberglaan 100, Utrecht 3584CX, The Netherlands
* Corresponding author.
E-mail address: f.barone@bham.ac.uk

Compelling evidence suggests that several biological processes can be involved in pSS and contribute to the establishment of salivary gland pathology. Those encompass pathways of activation belonging both to the innate and acquired immune systems, such as interferon (IFN) activation,[6] defective T-regulatory activity,[7] increased number and function of helper T cell (T_H) 17,[8] and excessive costimulation.[9,10] Lymphoneogenesis with germinal center (GC) formation and clonal expansion of malignant B cells is ascribed to the aberrant B-cell activation that characterized a subset of patients with high serum level of autoantibodies, systemic manifestations, and high risk of lymphoma development.[11]

Whether those pathogenic processes coexist in the same patient and manifest in different disease phases or whether different pathogenic processes occur in different subjects still represents an area of debate.

SALIVARY GLAND EPITHELIAL CELLS AND ACTIVATION OF THE INTERFERON TYPE I PATHWAY

The cross talk between salivary gland epithelial cells (SGECs) and the recruited lymphocytes plays a central role in salivary gland pathology. Some of the viruses and bacteria that display specific epithelial tropism have been implicated in SS pathogenesis.[12,13] Although a single responsible agent has not been identified, there are reports of viral involvement in support of the persistent antigenic exposure to locally recruited lymphocytes. Evidence of Epstein-Barr virus, cytomegalovirus, human herpesvirus type 6, human T-lymphotropic virus type I, human herpesvirus type 8, and coxsackie virus infection have been provided in pSS.[14]

Pathogen-induced SGEC damage is deemed responsible for the release of autoantigens and induction of intrinsic mechanisms of cellular responses.[15,16] It is believed that critical modifications of the SGEC expression profiles occur on injury and that SGECs isolated from pSS patients can maintain those changes in vitro.[17] Toll-like receptor (TLR) engagement, in particular TLR3 for SGECs and TLR7 and TLR8 for plasmacytoid dendritic cells (pDCs), is involved in the earliest phases of pSS pathology.[18] This results in local up-regulation of the type I IFN genes in both SGECs and pDCs.[19,20] The importance of type I INF activation is further supported by the association between IRF5 and STAT4 polymorphisms with disease susceptibility.[21] Locally released IFN stimulates autocrine and paracrine release of the B cell activating factor (BAFF)[22] that, in turn, induces B-cell activation and supports autoantibody production and formation of immune complexes that stimulate recruited pDCs[23] for the further release of IFN.[24] The presence of the risk alleles for IRF5 correlates with a high level of *IRF5* mRNA in both peripheral blood mononuclear cells and SGECs and with increased levels of IFN-induced gene transcripts.[25] Similarly, STAT4 activation is responsible for the IL-12–dependent activation of natural killer (NK) cells, polarization of naïve $CD4^+$ T cells to IFN-γ producing T_H1 cells, and the IL-23–dependent expansion of T_H17 cells,[26] thus dramatically contributing to the autoimmune process.

The pathogenic cross talk established in the earliest phases of pSS between leukocytes and SGECs is maintained during the length of the disease. SGECs provide key signals that enable recruitment (CCL17, CCL19, CCL21, CCL22, CXCL10, CXCL12, and CXCL13[3,27,28]) and adhesion molecules that facilitate the organization of the lymphocytic aggregates and are responsible for the classical periductal distribution of the foci.

To the recruited lymphocytes, SGECs provide survival factors and antigen presentation. SGECs release autoantigens in apoptotic blebs[29] or in actively secreted vesicles.[15] Direct presentation of nuclear extractable proteins, such as Ro52, which correlates with salivary inflammation,[30] in association with the up-regulated MHC-II[31] and in complex with CD40 has also been described.[32]

SGECs are also responsible for the production of T-cell homeostatic cytokines, such as IL-7 and thymic stromal lymphopoietin (TSLP). IL-7 is a key mediator of salivary gland T-cell activation[33,34]; it is released on TLR activation[34,35] and its levels correlate with the focus score (number of periductal foci in 4 mm^2)[36] and the total number of infiltrating T cells.[33] An increased number of IL-7R cells is found in the salivary glands of pSS patients compared with sicca patients.[37] Finally, ectopic IL-7 contributes to IFN-γ–mediated T$_H$1 response and the formation of T$_H$17.[38,39] In contrast to IL-7, TSLP is decreased in pSS patients' salivary glands and TSLP expression negatively correlates with T-cell infiltration and markers of inflammation. As such, TSLP seems to function as a mediator in tissue homeostasis.[40] As discussed previously, SGECs express BAFF,[22] which is a critical factor in B-cell activation and survival.[24,41]

The ectopic production of lymphocyte survival factors supports the expansion and persistence within the glands of autoreactive clones, naturally deemed to die for the scarce expression of follicle-associated chemokine receptors (such as CXCR5) and BAFF receptor.[42] Not surprisingly, the serum expression of those cytokines correlates significantly with local expansion and organization of the lymphocytic aggregates, with markers of disease activity and autoantibody production, thus providing a promising therapeutic target in pSS.[43]

T LYMPHOCYTES

The composition of the lymphocytic infiltration of the salivary gland is dependent on the grade of infiltration and inflammation. Small lymphocytic foci, organized around the intralobular and interlobular ducts[36,44,45] mainly consist of CD4$^+$ T cells and dendritic cells. Progressive increase of the B-cell component is observed, during the disease course, which correlates with onset of systemic manifestations and increased focus score.[45] Formation of germinal centers (GCs), areas of lymphocyte proliferation within the dense packed B-cell infiltrate, is observed in approximately 20% to 25% of SS patients.[2] More common is the presence of organized foci, with separate T-cell or B-cell rich areas, in absence of fully formed GCs.[3]

Although the potential viral etiology and the predominance of the type I IFN response suggest a predominance of CD8$^+$ T cells, CD4$^+$ cells embody the majority of infiltrating T lymphocytes. CD8$^+$ T cells are present in pSS infiltrates[45] but at relatively low numbers and are not considered to play a major part in pathogenesis.

Salivary gland infiltrating CD4$^+$ T cells display an activated phenotype[45] and contribute to disease pathogenesis, both releasing pathogenic cytokines and providing support to recruited B cells. CD4$^+$ cell-derived cytokines are mainly represented by IFN-γ and interleukin (IL)-17, which are associated with salivary gland tissue damage.[8,29] IFN-γ is produced both by T cells and NK cells and is involved in epithelial cell activation, promoting antimicrobial protection, apoptosis, inflammation, and tissue damage by up-regulation of IFN II-induced genes.[9,29,46,47] In the periphery, up-regulated IFN-inducible genes (IFN signature, both types I and II) are found in approximately 50% of SS patients, as reviewed elsewhere.[48]

The presence of a type I IFN signature has been associated with a more severe disease phenotype, including a higher European League Against Rheumatism Sjögren's Syndrome Disease Activity Index score, increased autoantibody production, and hypergammaglobulinemia.[6] Nonetheless, a recent study demonstrated that in patients with high salivary gland expression of IFN-inducible genes, patients could be divided in groups with type I, type II, and mixed predominance, with the type II predominance associated with higher focus score and increased lymphoma risk.[46,49] Stratifying the patients according to the type of IFN predominance might provide an interesting tool for disease prognosis and response to treatment.

The authors' group has recently demonstrated that in an animal model of pSS, infiltrating T cells also produce IL-22, a mucosa-associated homeostatic cytokine involved in epithelial response to damage.[50] Aberrant salivary gland expression of IL-22 enables the ectopic production of the lymphoid chemokines CXCL13 and CXCL12, respectively, by fibroblasts and epithelial cells, thus contributing to lymphocyte organization and GC formation.[50] In pSS, T_H17 and $NKp44^+$ NK cells represent the major cellular source of IL-22.[51]

Although increasing evidence shows involvement of T_H2 activity in the salivary glands, the exact contribution of T_H2 cytokines is unclear. A correlation between the degree of local inflammation and a bias toward a T_H1-predominant infiltrate has been made.[52] Nonetheless, significant increase in T_H2 cytokines is observed in GC-positive patients.[53] The authors' group previously demonstrated the association between IL-18, a known cytokine involved in the T_H1/T_H2 switch, with the increased production of antibodies against ENA.[54] Another cytokine, IL-21, involved in T_H17 cell homeostasis, plasma cells differentiation, and GC formation, is found in pSS salivary glands. Its expression correlates with IgG1 levels, anti-Ro/SSA antibody titters, and the degree of lymphocytic infiltration.[55] In pSS patients, an increase in number of both circulating and salivary gland IL-21^+ T follicular helper cells correlates with the number of memory B cells and plasma cells.[56,57]

CD4-CD8 double-negative T cells have also been reported to infiltrate the salivary glands, at later stages of disease; those are associated with the symptoms of dryness and presence of GC-like structures in the salivary glands.[58]

B CELLS AND LYMPHONEOGENESIS

Progressive B-cell aggregation in the salivary glands is mediated by the aberrant production of the B-cell chemoattractant CXCL13, derived from SGECs,[5] IL-22–activated stromal cells,[50] and macrophages.[3,59] Alongside CXCL13, ectopic expression of CCL21, CCL19, and CXCL12 has been described in the salivary glands of pSS patients and animal models of the disease.[3,60,61] The expression of these lymphoid chemokines, responsible for recruitment, positioning, and degree of organization of B and T compartments, can be detected in discrete areas within ectopic lymphoid structures, resembling the lymphoid organization observed in secondary lymphoid organs (SLOs).[3] Increased gene expression of those chemokines and their receptors correlates with B-cell accumulation and presence of GC in pSS salivary glands.[62]

In a high proportion of pSS patients, the B cells present within salivary gland GCs lack the markers commonly found in typical GC B cells, such as CD10 and CD38.[63] A small percentage of pSS patients (approximately 5%) presents with $CD21^+$ $CD38^+$ B cells in the lymphoid infiltrates, consistent with the phenotype observed in chronically activated tonsillar GC B cells.[64] Still, most B cells found in the salivary glands of pSS patients display a phenotype consistent with Transitional type 2 B cells, a mature subset of transitional B cells, and marginal zone–type B cells ($CD19^+$ IgD^+ $CD38-IgM^+$ $CD21^+$ $CD23^+$ and $CD20^+$ IgD^+ $CD38-CD21^+$ $CD24^+$).[63,65,66] Recently, $CD138^+$ $Bcl-2^+$ plasma cells have been detected in areas characterized by CXCL12 and IL-6 expression in pSS salivary glands with high focus score.[67] Moreover, the presence of anti-Ro/SSA and anti-La/SSB (whose serum detection is an important diagnostic criteria)–producing cells has been described in the periphery of GC-like structures in labial salivary gland biopsies.[2,68] Increasing interest has been raised on the ability of B cells to contribute to the development of autoimmunity, specifically the ability of B cells to regulate dendritic cells, activate T cells, act as antigen-presenting cells, and secrete cytokines.[69,70]

The cross talk between T cells and B cells is of paramount importance for the generation of the GC reaction. GC-like structures can be identified in salivary gland histologic sections and their presence correlates with higher focus score and extensive B-cell infiltration.[71] Histologically, GCs can be identified as areas of lighter staining (due to the presence of lymphoblasts and follicular dendritic cell networks) within darker confined and organized areas of active B-cell proliferation mainly populated by centroblasts.[2] In minor salivary glands, segregation into dark and light zone compartments is not as easily identified as in major glands. Sensitivity in the detection can be enhanced by CD21, CD23, bcl-6, and CD35 stainings.[72] GCs, both in minor and major salivary glands, host the machinery that enables the process of B-cell affinity maturation. The presence of the enzyme activation-induced cytidine deaminase (AID) has been described by the authors' group within GC-positive pSS salivary glands.[60]

The possible association between ectopic GC formation and the development of B-cell lymphoma (observed in 3.4%–7% of pSS patients[73–75]) had been long suspected on the basis of the biological risk related to clonal cell expansion at ectopic sites. In SLOs, the direction of travel of lymphocytes is established by stringent gradients of chemokine expression and resident stromal cells set the availability of locally released survival factors.[76] Lymphocyte survival and proliferation in SLO is also controlled by the access to the follicles and limited by the competition between alloreactive and autoreactive clones (that present down-regulated CXCR5 and BAFF receptor expression).[42] In the salivary glands, the ability to screen autoreactive clones is doubtful in GCs that lack a rigorous anatomic segregation. Although a process of progressive transformation of the resident salivary glands stroma toward lymphoid stroma has been described,[50] this does not seem to reproduce the degree of organization present in SLO GCs. Expression of CXCL13 is not confined within the B-cell area; the expression of CCL21 is limited to the perivascular myofibroblasts and aberrant niches for B aggregation are provided by locally activated SGECs.[3,77] This "confusing" microenvironment for lymphocyte migration is accompanied by aberrant and diffuse expression of BAFF and a proliferation-inducing ligand (APRIL) that enables survival of autoreactive, pathogenic clones that in SLOs would be classically excluded from the follicles. It is, therefore, not surprising that somehow GC formation is associated with lymphoma development. Theander and colleagues,[11] however, could not establish a positive correlation between the 2 histologic entities (14%) but did define a strong negative correlation between the absence of GC detection and the nondevelopment of B-cell lymphoma,[2,60] supporting the concept that uncontrolled B-cell clonal expansion represents a critical step in lymphomagenesis. Nonetheless, a more rigorous characterization of the additional stages involved in lymphomagenesis is needed to better understand this phenomenon.

In this context, it is important to highlight the largely unexplored pathogenic cross talk between the GC and the areas of lymphoepithelial proliferation within the lymphoepithelial sialoadenitis (LESA). Large areas of LESA are commonly considered to be premalignant lesions in inflamed glands. Within established samples of MALT lymphoma, malignant B cells that bear histological features of immunoblasts or centroblasts are preferentially distributed in sheets. These sheets either infiltrate the reactive follicles, assuming the characteristic marginal one distribution, or, more often, spread in the interfollicular area adjacent to the LESA.[77,78] A clonal relationship between the polyclonal B-cell expansion occurring within the GC of pSS patients and the following lymphomatous transformation has been established; however, the role of epithelial cells and the pathogenic relevance of LESA/GC interaction during lymphomagenesis should be further exploited.

TISSUE DAMAGE/FIBROSIS AND DRYNESS

The cardinal sign of pSS is dryness; on the other hand, the focal lymphocytic infiltration represents the hallmark histopathologic finding of the disease. Correlations have been made between the extent of the lymphocytic infiltrate (focus score) and salivary gland function; however, to date the contribution of SGEC dysfunction, tissue destruction, autoantibody production, and fibrosis to oral dryness is not clear. An association between fibrosis and saliva production has also been reported[79] and, finally, a potential role for dysregulated neuroendocrine mechanisms has to be taken into consideration.[80] Thus, multiple pathogenic components could contribute to oral dryness and further studies are needed to dissect their relative weight.

SUMMARY

The salivary glands provide the hub of pSS pathology. Pathogenic processes have been identified that contribute to disease establishment and progression; nonetheless, several areas remain unexplored. The possibility of using process-driven stratification in pSS, the potential identification of biological fingerprints associated with disease phases, and the biological cross talk responsible for lymphoma development and functional damage remain to be addressed. As such, pSS remains a fascinating disease to study with significant unmet clinical need.

REFERENCES

1. Fox RI. Sjogren's syndrome. Lancet 2005;366(9482):321–31.
2. Salomonsson S, Jonsson MV, Skarstein K, et al. Cellular basis of ectopic germinal center formation and autoantibody production in the target organ of patients with Sjogren's syndrome. Arthritis Rheum 2003;48(11):3187–201.
3. Barone F, Bombardieri M, Manzo A, et al. Association of CXCL13 and CCL21 expression with the progressive organization of lymphoid-like structures in Sjogren's syndrome. Arthritis Rheum 2005;52(6):1773–84.
4. Mariette X. Therapeutic potential for B-cell modulation in Sjogren's syndrome. Rheum Dis Clin North Am 2008;34(4):1025–33, x.
5. Amft N, Curnow SJ, Scheel-Toellner D, et al. Ectopic expression of the B cell-attracting chemokine BCA-1 (CXCL13) on endothelial cells and within lymphoid follicles contributes to the establishment of germinal center-like structures in Sjogren's syndrome. Arthritis Rheum 2001;44(11):2633–41.
6. Brkic Z, Maria NI, van Helden-Meeuwsen CG, et al. Prevalence of interferon type I signature in CD14 monocytes of patients with Sjogren's syndrome and association with disease activity and BAFF gene expression. Ann Rheum Dis 2013; 72(5):728–35.
7. Christodoulou MI, Kapsogeorgou EK, Moutsopoulos NM, et al. Foxp3+ T-regulatory cells in Sjogren's syndrome: correlation with the grade of the autoimmune lesion and certain adverse prognostic factors. Am J Pathol 2008;173(5):1389–96.
8. Katsifis GE, Rekka S, Moutsopoulos NM, et al. Systemic and local interleukin-17 and linked cytokines associated with Sjogren's syndrome immunopathogenesis. Am J Pathol 2009;175(3):1167–77.
9. Dimitriou ID, Kapsogeorgou EK, Moutsopoulos HM, et al. CD40 on salivary gland epithelial cells: high constitutive expression by cultured cells from Sjogren's

syndrome patients indicating their intrinsic activation. Clin Exp Immunol 2002; 127(2):386–92.

10. Gong YZ, Nitiham J, Taylor K, et al. Differentiation of follicular helper T cells by salivary gland epithelial cells in primary Sjogren's syndrome. J autoimmun 2014;51:57–66.

11. Theander E, Vasaitis L, Baecklund E, et al. Lymphoid organisation in labial salivary gland biopsies is a possible predictor for the development of malignant lymphoma in primary Sjogren's syndrome. Ann Rheum Dis 2011;70(8):1363–8.

12. Lugonja B, Yeo L, Milward MR, et al. Periodontitis prevalence and serum antibody reactivity to periodontal bacteria in primary Sjogren's syndrome: a pilot study. J Clin Periodontol 2016;43:26–33.

13. Lucchesi D, Pitzalis C, Bombardieri M. EBV and other viruses as triggers of tertiary lymphoid structures in primary Sjogren's syndrome. Expert Rev Clin Immunol 2014;10(4):445–55.

14. Kivity S, Arango MT, Ehrenfeld M, et al. Infection and autoimmunity in Sjogren's syndrome: a clinical study and comprehensive review. J Autoimmun 2014;51:17–22.

15. Kapsogeorgou EK, Abu-Helu RF, Moutsopoulos HM, et al. Salivary gland epithelial cell exosomes: a source of autoantigenic ribonucleoproteins. Arthritis Rheum 2005;52(5):1517–21.

16. Manoussakis MN, Kapsogeorgou EK. The role of epithelial cells in the pathogenesis of Sjogren's syndrome. Clin Rev Allergy Immunol 2007;32(3):225–30.

17. Fox RI, Kang HI, Ando D, et al. Cytokine mRNA expression in salivary gland biopsies of Sjogren's syndrome. J Immunol 1994;152(11):5532–9.

18. Kawakami A, Nakashima K, Tamai M, et al. Toll-like receptor in salivary glands from patients with Sjogren's syndrome: functional analysis by human salivary gland cell line. J Rheumatol 2007;34(5):1019–26.

19. Gottenberg JE, Cagnard N, Lucchesi C, et al. Activation of IFN pathways and plasmacytoid dendritic cell recruitment in target organs of primary Sjogren's syndrome. Proc Natl Acad Sci U S A 2006;103(8):2770–5.

20. Zhao J, Kubo S, Nakayamada S, et al. Association of plasmacytoid dendritic cells with B cell infiltration in minor salivary glands in patients with Sjogren's syndrome. Mod Rheumatol 2015;1–9.

21. Nordmark G, Kristjansdottir G, Theander E, et al. Additive effects of the major risk alleles of IRF5 and STAT4 in primary Sjogren's syndrome. Genes Immun 2009; 10(1):68–76.

22. Ittah M, Miceli-Richard C, Gottenberg JE, et al. Viruses induce high expression of BAFF by salivary gland epithelial cells through TLR- and type-I IFN-dependent and -independent pathways. Eur J Immunol 2008;38(4):1058–64.

23. Wildenberg ME, van Helden-Meeuwsen CG, van de Merwe JP, et al. Systemic increase in type I interferon activity in Sjogren's syndrome: a putative role for plasmacytoid dendritic cells. Eur J Immunol 2008;38(7):2024–33.

24. Ittah M, Miceli-Richard C, Lebon P, et al. Induction of B cell-activating factor by viral infection is a general phenomenon, but the types of viruses and mechanisms depend on cell type. J Innate Immun 2011;3(2):200–7.

25. Miceli-Richard C, Gestermann N, Ittah M, et al. The CGGGG insertion/deletion polymorphism of the IRF5 promoter is a strong risk factor for primary Sjogren's syndrome. Arthritis Rheum 2009;60(7):1991–7.

26. Frucht DM, Aringer M, Galon J, et al. Stat4 is expressed in activated peripheral blood monocytes, dendritic cells, and macrophages at sites of Th1-mediated inflammation. J Immunol 2000;164(9):4659–64.

27. Xanthou G, Polihronis M, Tzioufas AG, et al. "Lymphoid" chemokine messenger RNA expression by epithelial cells in the chronic inflammatory lesion of the salivary glands of Sjogren's syndrome patients: possible participation in lymphoid structure formation. Arthritis Rheum 2001;44(2):408–18.

28. Moriyama M, Hayashida JN, Toyoshima T, et al. Cytokine/chemokine profiles contribute to understanding the pathogenesis and diagnosis of primary Sjogren's syndrome. Clin Exp Immunol 2012;169(1):17–26.

29. Abu-Helu RF, Dimitriou ID, Kapsogeorgou EK, et al. Induction of salivary gland epithelial cell injury in Sjogren's syndrome: in vitro assessment of T cell-derived cytokines and Fas protein expression. J Autoimmun 2001;17(2):141–53.

30. Aqrawi LA, Kvarnström M, Brokstad KA, et al. Ductal epithelial expression of Ro52 correlates with inflammation in salivary glands of patients with primary Sjogren's syndrome. Clin Exp Immunol 2014;177(1):244–52.

31. Nakken B, Jonsson R, Brokstad KA, et al. Associations of MHC class II alleles in Norwegian primary Sjogren's syndrome patients: implications for development of autoantibodies to the Ro52 autoantigen. Scand J Immunol 2001;54(4):428–33.

32. Nakamura H, Kawakami A, Tominaga M, et al. Expression of CD40/CD40 ligand and Bcl-2 family proteins in labial salivary glands of patients with Sjogren's syndrome. Lab Invest 1999;79(3):261–9.

33. Bikker A, van Woerkom JM, Kruize AA, et al. Increased expression of interleukin-7 in labial salivary glands of patients with primary Sjogren's syndrome correlates with increased inflammation. Arthritis Rheum 2010;62(4):969–77.

34. Jin JO, Shinohara Y, Yu Q. Innate immune signaling induces interleukin-7 production from salivary gland cells and accelerates the development of primary Sjogren's syndrome in a mouse model. PLoS One 2013;8(10):e77605.

35. Jin JO, Kawai T, Cha S, et al. Interleukin-7 enhances the Th1 response to promote the development of Sjogren's syndrome-like autoimmune exocrinopathy in mice. Arthritis Rheum 2013;65(8):2132–42.

36. Chisholm DM, Mason DK. Labial salivary gland biopsy in Sjogren's disease. J Clin Pathol 1968;21(5):656–60.

37. Bikker A, Kruize AA, Wenting M, et al. Increased interleukin (IL)-7Ralpha expression in salivary glands of patients with primary Sjogren's syndrome is restricted to T cells and correlates with IL-7 expression, lymphocyte numbers and activity. Ann Rheum Dis 2012;71(6):1027–33.

38. Lee H, Park HJ, Sohn HJ, et al. Combinatorial therapy for liver metastatic colon cancer: dendritic cell vaccine and low-dose agonistic anti-4-1BB antibody costimulatory signal. J Surg Res 2011;169(1):e43–50.

39. Pellegrini P, Contasta I, Del Beato T, et al. Gender-specific cytokine pathways, targets, and biomarkers for the switch from health to adenoma and colorectal cancer. Clin Dev Immunol 2011;2011:819724.

40. Hillen MR, Kruize AA, Bikker A, et al. Decreased expression of thymic stromal lymphopoietin in salivary glands of patients with primary Sjogren's syndrome is associated with increased disease activity. Mod Rheumatol 2016;26(1):105–9.

41. Roescher N, Vosters JL, Alsaleh G, et al. Targeting the splicing of mRNA in autoimmune diseases: BAFF inhibition in Sjogren's syndrome as a proof of concept. Mol Ther 2014;22(4):821–7.

42. Ekland EH, Forster R, Lipp M, et al. Requirements for follicular exclusion and competitive elimination of autoantigen-binding B cells. J Immunol 2004;172(8):4700–8.

43. Mariette X, Seror R, Quartuccio L, et al. Efficacy and safety of belimumab in primary Sjogren's syndrome: results of the BELISS open-label phase II study. Ann Rheum Dis 2015;74(3):526–31.

44. Greenspan JS, Daniels TE, Talal N, et al. The histopathology of Sjogren's syndrome in labial salivary gland biopsies. Oral Surg Oral Med Oral Pathol 1974; 37(2):217–29.
45. Christodoulou MI, Kapsogeorgou EK, Moutsopoulos HM. Characteristics of the minor salivary gland infiltrates in Sjogren's syndrome. J Autoimmun 2010;34(4): 400–7.
46. Nezos A, Gravani F, Tassidou A, et al. Type I and II interferon signatures in Sjogren's syndrome pathogenesis: Contributions in distinct clinical phenotypes and Sjogren's related lymphomagenesis. J Autoimmun 2015;63:47–58.
47. van Woerkom JM, Kruize AA, Wenting-van Wijk MJ, et al. Salivary gland and peripheral blood T helper 1 and 2 cell activity in Sjogren's syndrome compared with non-Sjogren's sicca syndrome. Ann Rheum Dis 2005;64(10):1474–9.
48. Brkic Z, Versnel MA. Type I IFN signature in primary Sjogren's syndrome patients. Expert Rev Clin Immunol 2014;10(4):457–67.
49. Hall JC, Baer AN, Shah AA, et al. Molecular Subsetting of Interferon Pathways in Sjogren's Syndrome. Arthritis Rheumatol 2015;67(9):2437–46.
50. Barone F, Nayar S, Campos J, et al. IL-22 regulates lymphoid chemokine production and assembly of tertiary lymphoid organs. Proc Natl Acad Sci U S A 2015; 112(35):11024–9.
51. Ciccia F, Guggino G, Rizzo A, et al. Potential involvement of IL-22 and IL-22-producing cells in the inflamed salivary glands of patients with Sjogren's syndrome. Ann Rheum Dis 2012;71(2):295–301.
52. Mitsias DI, Tzioufas AG, Veiopoulou C, et al. The Th1/Th2 cytokine balance changes with the progress of the immunopathological lesion of Sjogren's syndrome. Clin Exp Immunol 2002;128(3):562–8.
53. Maehara T, Moriyama M, Hayashida JN, et al. Selective localization of T helper subsets in labial salivary glands from primary Sjogren's syndrome patients. Clin Exp Immunol 2012;169(2):89–99.
54. Bombardieri M, Barone F, Pittoni V, et al. Increased circulating levels and salivary gland expression of interleukin-18 in patients with Sjogren's syndrome: relationship with autoantibody production and lymphoid organization of the periductal inflammatory infiltrate. Arthritis Res Ther 2004;6(5):R447–56.
55. Kang EH, Lee YJ, Hyon JY, et al. Salivary cytokine profiles in primary Sjogren's syndrome differ from those in non-Sjogren sicca in terms of TNF-alpha levels and Th-1/Th-2 ratios. Clin Exp Rheumatol 2011;29(6):970–6.
56. Jin L, Yu D, Li X, et al. CD4+CXCR5+ follicular helper T cells in salivary gland promote B cells maturation in patients with primary Sjogren's syndrome. Int J Clin Exp Pathol 2014;7(5):1988–96.
57. Simpson N, Gatenby PA, Wilson A, et al. Expansion of circulating T cells resembling follicular helper T cells is a fixed phenotype that identifies a subset of severe systemic lupus erythematosus. Arthritis Rheum 2010;62(1):234–44.
58. Alunno A, Carubbi F, Bistoni O, et al. CD4(-)CD8(-) T-cells in primary Sjogren's syndrome: association with the extent of glandular involvement. J Autoimmun 2014;51:38–43.
59. Kramer JM, Klimatcheva E, Rothstein TL. CXCL13 is elevated in Sjogren's syndrome in mice and humans and is implicated in disease pathogenesis. J Leukoc Biol 2013;94(5):1079–89.
60. Bombardieri M, Barone F, Humby F, et al. Activation-induced cytidine deaminase expression in follicular dendritic cell networks and interfollicular large B cells supports functionality of ectopic lymphoid neogenesis in autoimmune sialoadenitis and MALT lymphoma in Sjogren's syndrome. J Immunol 2007;179(7):4929–38.

61. Bombardieri M, Barone F, Lucchesi D, et al. Inducible tertiary lymphoid structures, autoimmunity, and exocrine dysfunction in a novel model of salivary gland inflammation in C57BL/6 mice. J Immunol 2012;189(7):3767–76.

62. Carubbi F, Alunno A, Cipriani P, et al. Is minor salivary gland biopsy more than a diagnostic tool in primary Sjogrens syndrome? Association between clinical, histopathological, and molecular features: a retrospective study. Semin Arthritis Rheum 2014;44(3):314–24.

63. Youinou P, Devauchelle-Pensec V, Pers JO. Significance of B cells and B cell clonality in Sjogren's syndrome. Arthritis Rheum 2010;62(9):2605–10.

64. Johnsen SJ, Berget E, Jonsson MV, et al. Evaluation of germinal center-like structures and B cell clonality in patients with primary Sjogren syndrome with and without lymphoma. J Rheumatol 2014;41(11):2214–22.

65. Youinou P, Pers JO. The late news on baff in autoimmune diseases. Autoimmun Rev 2010;9(12):804–6.

66. Le Pottier L, Devauchelle V, Fautrel A, et al. Ectopic germinal centers are rare in Sjogren's syndrome salivary glands and do not exclude autoreactive B cells. J Immunol 2009;182(6):3540–7.

67. Szyszko EA, Brokstad KA, Oijordsbakken G, et al. Salivary glands of primary Sjogren's syndrome patients express factors vital for plasma cell survival. Arthritis Res Ther 2011;13(1):R2.

68. Tengner P, Halse AK, Haga HJ, et al. Detection of anti-Ro/SSA and anti-La/SSB autoantibody-producing cells in salivary glands from patients with Sjogren's syndrome. Arthritis Rheum 1998;41(12):2238–48.

69. Youinou P, Saraux A, Pers JO. B-lymphocytes govern the pathogenesis of Sjogren's syndrome. Curr Pharm Biotechnol 2012;13(10):2071–7.

70. Jonsson R, Nginamau E, Szyszko E, et al. Role of B cells in Sjogren's syndrome–from benign lymphoproliferation to overt malignancy. Front Biosci 2007;12: 2159–70.

71. Risselada AP, Looije MF, Kruize AA, et al. The role of ectopic germinal centers in the immunopathology of primary Sjogren's syndrome: a systematic review. Semin Arthritis Rheum 2013;42(4):368–76.

72. Jonsson MV, Skarstein K. Follicular dendritic cells confirm lymphoid organization in the minor salivary glands of primary Sjogren's syndrome. J Oral Pathol Med 2008;37(9):515–21.

73. Voulgarelis M, Dafni UG, Isenberg DA, et al. Malignant lymphoma in primary Sjogren's syndrome: a multicenter, retrospective, clinical study by the European Concerted Action on Sjogren's Syndrome. Arthritis Rheum 1999;42(8):1765–72.

74. Sutcliffe N, Inanc M, Speight P, et al. Predictors of lymphoma development in primary Sjogren's syndrome. Semin Arthritis Rheum 1998;28(2):80–7.

75. Theander E, Henriksson G, Ljungberg O, et al. Lymphoma and other malignancies in primary Sjogren's syndrome: a cohort study on cancer incidence and lymphoma predictors. Ann Rheum Dis 2006;65(6):796–803.

76. Buckley CD, Barone F, Nayar S, et al. Stromal cells in chronic inflammation and tertiary lymphoid organ formation. Annu Rev Immunol 2015;33:715–45.

77. Barone F, Bombardieri M, Rosado MM, et al. CXCL13, CCL21, and CXCL12 expression in salivary glands of patients with Sjogren's syndrome and MALT lymphoma: association with reactive and malignant areas of lymphoid organization. J Immunol 2008;180(7):5130–40.

78. Isaacson PG, Wotherspoon AC, Diss T, et al. Follicular colonization in B-cell lymphoma of mucosa-associated lymphoid tissue. Am J Surg Pathol 1991;15(9): 819–28.

79. Bookman AA, Shen H, Cook RJ, et al. Whole stimulated salivary flow: correlation with the pathology of inflammation and damage in minor salivary gland biopsy specimens from patients with primary Sjogren's syndrome but not patients with sicca. Arthritis Rheum 2011;63(7):2014–20.

80. Tzioufas AG, Tsonis J, Moutsopoulos HM. Neuroendocrine dysfunction in Sjogren's syndrome. Neuroimmunomodulation 2008;15(1):37–45.

Parotid Gland Biopsy, the Alternative Way to Diagnose Sjögren Syndrome

 CrossMark

Fred K.L. Spijkervet, DMD, PhD[a],*, Erlin Haacke, MD[b,c],
Frans G.M. Kroese, PhD[b], Hendrika Bootsma, MD, PhD[b],
Arjan Vissink, DMD, MD, PhD[a]

KEYWORDS

- Sjögren syndrome • Parotid gland • Labial gland • Salivary gland • Biopsy
- Diagnostics

KEY POINTS

- In Sjögren diagnostics, parotid gland incision biopsies can overcome most disadvantages of minor salivary gland excision biopsies.
- Sensitivity and specificity of parotid and minor salivary gland biopsies for diagnosing Sjögren syndrome are comparable.
- Lymphoepithelial lesions and early stage lymphomas are easier to detect in parotid gland tissue of patients with Sjögren syndrome.
- In contrast to minor salivary glands, repeated biopsies of the same parotid gland are possible, which is an important asset in monitoring disease progression as well as in studying the efficacy of treatment at a glandular tissue level.
- Histopathologic results from the parotid gland can be compared with other diagnostic results derived from the same gland (sialometry sialochemistry, sialography, scintigraphy, ultrasound, computed tomography, MRI).

INTRODUCTION

Salivary gland biopsy is a technique broadly applied in the diagnostic work-up of Sjögren syndrome (SS) as well as lymphoma accompanying SS, sarcoidosis, amyloidosis, and other connective tissue disorders. A focus score of 1 or greater per 4 mm^2 labial

Disclosure Statement: The authors have nothing to disclose.
[a] Department of Oral and Maxillofacial Surgery, University of Groningen, University Medical Center Groningen, PO Box 30.001, 9700 RB Groningen, The Netherlands; [b] Department of Rheumatology and Clinical Immunology, University of Groningen, University Medical Center Groningen, PO Box 30.001, 9700 RB Groningen, The Netherlands; [c] Department of Pathology and Medical Biology, University of Groningen, University Medical Center Groningen, PO Box 30.001, 9700 RB Groningen, The Netherlands
* Corresponding author.
E-mail address: f.k.l.spijkervet@umcg.nl

salivary gland tissue is considered as one of the 4 objective European-American Consensus Group classification criteria (AECG)[1] and one of the 3 objective American College of Rheumatology (ACR) provisional classification criteria[2] for SS. The focus scores reflect the number of infiltrates of 50 or greater mononuclear inflammatory cells, predominantly lymphocytes, in a perivascular or periductal location, typically adjacent to normal acini, per 4 mm^2 salivary gland tissue.[3,4] Also in the under-construction consensus classification criteria of the European League against Rheumatism (EULAR) and ACR, a labial focus score of 1 or greater will be maintained as a leading classification criterion.[5]

Moreover, there are views that besides being of diagnostic value, labial salivary gland biopsies also may play a role in predicting lymphoma development[6] as well as in monitoring disease and treatment efficacy.[7–9] Recently, Fisher and colleagues[10] reviewed the labial salivary gland pathologic changes that characterizes SS. They concluded that labial salivary gland biopsies offer a distinct potential as a biomarker in primary SS (pSS), particularly relevant to glandular involvement, and offer additional prognostic, stratification, and mechanistic insights. They also added that precise value of a labial salivary gland biopsy is yet hard to determine in the absence of proven immunomodulatory therapies in pSS and that further work on validation and understanding the natural history is needed.

In their review, Fisher and colleagues[10] briefly mentioned parotid biopsies as an alternative to labial salivary gland biopsies but did not further state the advantages and disadvantages of parotid biopsies compared with labial salivary biopsies (**Table 1**).[11,12] In this contribution, the authors discuss the potential of parotid salivary gland biopsies as an alternative way to diagnose SS and also with emphasis of its added value in lymphoma diagnostics and rating disease progression and treatment efficacy.

MINOR SALIVARY GLAND BIOPSY

Minor salivary glands are widely distributed in the labial, buccal, and palatal mucosa of the oral cavity. Because pathognomonic changes are seen in minor salivary glands, labial salivary gland biopsy is largely used for assisting the diagnosis of SS.[4,13,14]

Surgical Considerations

Minor salivary glands, and labial salivary glands in particular, are easily accessible. The labial salivary glands lie above the muscle layer and branches of the mental nerve (labial sensory nerves) and are separated from the oral mucous membrane by a thin layer of fibrous connective tissue. Although the chance of excessive bleeding is minimal because the arterial supply to the lip lies deep, there is a serious hazard of sensory nerve injury, as the labial sensory nerves are closely associated to the minor salivary glands (**Fig. 1**).

Chisholm and Mason[3] introduced labial salivary gland biopsies in the diagnosis of SS.[3] The biopsies involve oral preparation of patients with local anesthetic infiltration followed by excising an ellipse of oral mucous membrane down to the muscle layer. The wound was closed with 4-0–gauge silk sutures, which were removed after 4 to 5 days. Ideally 6 to 8 minor glands are harvested and sent for histopathologic examination.

Several clinicians have revised the Chisholm and Mason technique. Currently, the approach of Greenspan and colleagues[13] and Daniels[14] is mostly applied (**Fig. 2**). This approach is described in detail on the Sjögren's International Collaborative Clinical Alliance Web site.[15] In short, the biopsy has to be performed through the mucosa of the lower lip that appears normal clinically. After applying local anesthetics, the lip is everted to expose the mucosa. Next, a 1.0- to 1.5-cm horizontal incision will be made to the right or left of the midline, approximately halfway between the vestibule and the vermilion border and halfway between the midline and the labial commissure. The lamina propria is bluntly dissected to release the minor salivary glands from the lamina propria beyond the incision and to bring them into the operating field. Approximately 7 minor salivary glands should be removed to provide a minimum gland section area of 8 to 12 mm^2 for microscopic focus scoring.[10] Finally, the mucosal incision margins are repositioned and sutured with 5-0 rapid absorbable (polyglactin/L-lactide acid) sutures (see **Fig. 2**).

Histologic Grading

The first grading system for salivary gland biopsies was used by Chisholm and Mason[3] in an attempt to standardize the examined area and record the degree of histopathologic change. At present, according to the revised AECG and provisional ACR classification criteria for SS (and also in the recent ACR-EULAR classification under construction), a labial salivary gland biopsy is considered positive if the glands (obtained through normal-appearing mucosa) demonstrate focal lymphocytic sialadenitis, evaluated by an expert histopathologist, with a focus score of 1 or greater (**Fig. 3**). Diagnosis of nonspecific chronic sialadenitis, sclerosing chronic sialadenitis, and granulomatous inflammation need to be excluded. A sufficient area of labial salivary gland tissue has to be examined, as Al-Hashimi and colleagues[16] showed that focus score might differ on multiple sections taken from the same labial glands specimen.

Complications

Complications of labial salivary gland biopsies include localized (permanent) sensory alteration of the lip, external hematoma, local swelling, formation of granulomas, internal scarring and cheloid formation, failing sutures, and local pain.[11,13,14,17–24] The localized sensory alterations are frequently described with the terms *anesthesia*, *reduced* or *partial loss of sensation*, *transitory numbness*, and *hypoesthesia*. These localized sensory alterations of the vermillion border of the lower lip mucosa may last for a few months but can be permanent in up to 10%, which should be considered as relatively high for a diagnostic procedure.[11,18]

PAROTID GLAND BIOPSY

The parotid gland is divided into a superficial and deep lobe based on the course of the facial nerve as it passes through (see **Fig. 1**). The technique of the parotid gland biopsy was initially described by Kraaijenhagen[25] and modified by Pijpe and colleagues[11] (**Fig. 4**). The parotid biopsy is performed in the superficial lobe area where the facial nerve is 1.5 to 2 cm below the surface of the gland.

Surgical Considerations

In short, the area in the region of the earlobe is anesthetized (auriculotemporal nerve) with 0.5 mL local infiltration anesthesia followed by skin disinfection and standard preparation. With a No. 15 knife-blade, a small 1- to 2-cm incision is made just below the earlobe near the posterior border of the mandible. The skin is incised; after blunt dissection of the subdermal tissue, the parotid capsule is exposed, followed by carefully opening the capsule and excision of the required amount of superficial parotid gland tissue for histopathologic review. The capsule of the parotid gland and subcutaneous layer is closed with 5-0 absorbable (polyglycolic acid) sutures, whereas the skin is closed with 5-0 nylon sutures (see **Fig. 4**). With this surgical approach, there are no reports of development of sialoceles or fistula. For details see the instructional film.

Table 1
Techniques to perform a labial or parotid salivary gland biopsy

	Technique	Advantages	Complications
Labial gland			
Chisholm & Mason,[3] 1968	Ellipse of oral mucous membrane down to the muscle layer; harvest of 6–8 glands; wound closure with 4-0 silk sutures which must be removed after 4–5 d	• Widely distributed glands • Easily accessible glands • Minimal chance of bleeding • Can identify germinal center–like structures	• Localized, 6%–10% permanent, sensory alteration of the lips and skin in the mental region • Internal scarring and cheloid formation • Suture failing
Greenspan et al,[13] 1974	1.5–2.0 cm linear incision of mucosa, parallel to the vermillion border and lateral to the midline		
Marx et al,[18] 1988	Mucosal incision of 3.0 × 0.75 cm		
Delgado & Mosqueda,[19] 1989	Longitudinal incision of 1 cm in the labial mucosa in front of the mandibular cuspids		
Guevara-Gutierrez et al,[58] 2001	Punch biopsy		
Mahlstedt et al,[20] 2002	1.0- to 1.5-cm wedge-shaped incision between the midline and commissure		
Gorson & Ropper,[59] 2003	1-cm vertical incision just behind the wet line through the mucosa and submucosa		
Berquin et al,[21] 2006	Oblique incision, starting 1.5 cm from the midline and proceeding latero-inferiorly, avoiding the glandular free zone in the center of the lower lip		
Caporali et al,[22] 2007	Small incision of 2–3 mm on the inner surface of the lower lip		

Parotid gland			
Kraaijenhagen,[25] 1975 Marx et al,[18] 1988 McGuirt et al,[60] 2002 Baurmash,[61] 2005 Pijpe et al,[11] 2007	1- to 2-cm incision just below and behind the earlobe near the posterior angle of the mandible; skin is incised and the parotid capsule exposed by blunt dissection capsule of the gland opened and adequate amount of superficial parotid tissue removed, approximately 5 × 5 mm; procedure completed with a 2- to 3-layered closure	• Presence of germinal centers • Presence of LELs • (Early) identification of MALT • Can repeatedly harvest same gland • Direct comparison with other diagnostic results derived from the same gland (eg, secretory function, sialography, scintigraphy, ultrasound)	• Temporary change in sensory sensation of the skin in the area of the incision • More demanding surgical expertise
Adam et al,[62] 1992 Berquin et al,[21] 2006	Mucosal incision 1 cm anterolaterally from the Wharton duct to 1 cm anteroposterior; blunt dissection and harvest of 0.5 cm^3 of glandular tissue; wound edges joined with 1–2 resorbable stiches		

Abbreviations: LELs, lymphoepithelial lesions; MALT, mucosa-associated lymphoid tissue.

Adapted from Delli K, Haacke EA, Pollard RP, et al. Baseline characteristics of parotid gland histopatholology predict responsiveness of patients with primary Sjögren's syndrome to rituximab treatment. Scand J Immunol 2015;81(5):434–5.

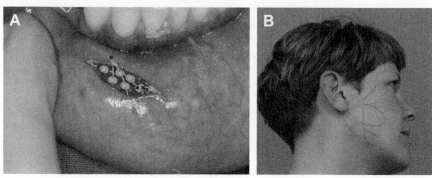

Fig. 1. Association of the labial and parotid salivary glands with, respectively, the mental and facial nerve. (*A*) The mental nerve (*) has 3 branches: one branch supplying the skin of the chin and 2 branches supplying the skin and mucous membrane of the lower lip. The branch that supplies the mucous membrane usually has 2 sub-branches of which the vertical one has an ascending course toward the vermillion border and is in close relation to the labial salivary glands (**). (*B*) The facial nerve enters the parotid gland forming a characteristic branching pattern that resembles a goose foot and is known as the pes anserinus. The parotid gland is divided into a superficial and deep lobe based on the course of the facial nerve as it passes through. In the area of the incisional biopsy of the parotid gland, the distance between the surface of the parotid gland and the facial nerve is approximately 1.5 to 2.0 cm. (*From* Delli K, Vissink A, Spijkervet FK. Salivary gland biopsy for Sjögren's syndrome. Oral Maxillofac Surg Clin North Am 2014;26(1):23–33; with permission.)

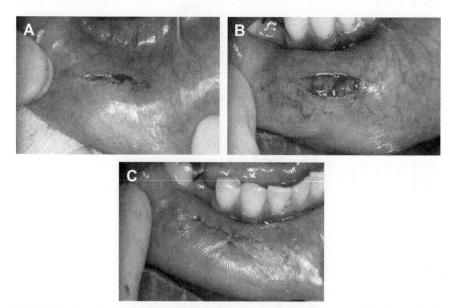

Fig. 2. Technique for harvesting labial salivary glands after infiltration of local anesthesia. (*A*) A horizontal incision of approximately 1.0 to 1.5 cm is made on the mucosal site of the lip. Just the epithelium is incised. (*B*) About 6 to 8 labial salivary glands are harvested avoiding damage to the branches of the mental nerve. (*C*) Wound closure with 5-0 rapid absorbable (polyglactin/ʟ-lactide acid) sutures; inverted buried notches.

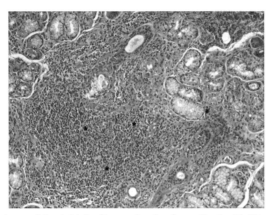

Fig. 3. Histopathology of the labial salivary glands of a patient with SS, which is characterized by lymphocytic infiltration (*asterisk*) of the excretory ducts and destruction of the acini, fulfilling the criterion of a focus score of 1 or greater (hematoxylin-eosin, original magnification ×10).

Histologic Grading

Pijpe and colleagues[11] established a new set of validated histopathologic criteria for diagnosing SS in accordance with the AECG classification criteria based on biopsy of the parotid gland (**Fig. 5**). A parotid biopsy is considered positive when it has a focus

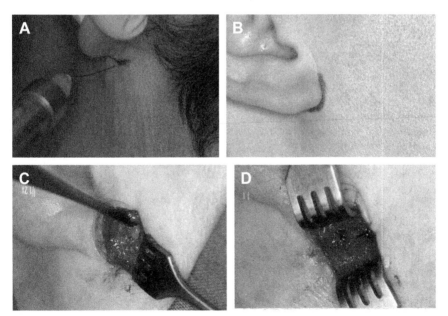

Fig. 4. Technique of a parotid biopsy. (*A*) The skin below the ear lobe is infiltrated with local anesthesia. (*B*) With a No. 15 blade a small 1- to 2-cm incision is made just below and behind the earlobe near the posterior border of the ascending ramus of the mandible. (*C*) The parotid capsule is exposed by blunt dissection after the skin incision. The capsule of the gland is carefully opened and a small amount of 5 × 5 × 5-mm superficial parotid tissue is removed. (*D*) The procedure is completed with a 2- to 3-layered closure with 4-0–gauge absorbable sutures (polyglycolic acid), while the skin layer is closed with 5-0 nylon sutures.

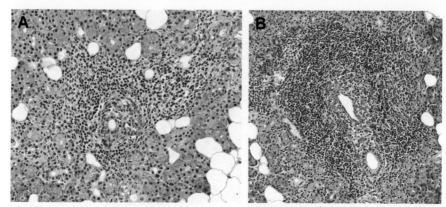

Fig. 5. Histopathology of the parotid salivary glands of a patient with SS. (*A*) Foci. (*B*) Lymphoepithelial lesions (H&E).

score of 1 or greater, defined as the number of lymphocytic foci (which are adjacent to normal-appearing acini and contain >50 lymphocytes) per 4 mm^2 of glandular parotid tissue (including fat tissue; see **Fig. 5**A), irrespective of the presence of benign lymphoepithelial lesions (LELs; see **Fig. 5**B). LELs are a characteristic histologic feature of the salivary, predominantly parotid, glands of patients with SS. LELs form through basal cell hyperplasia forming a multilayered epithelium. Between these reactive ductal epithelial cells, lymphocytes are present.

Complications

Potential complications of parotid salivary gland biopsies include the development of sialoceles and salivary fistulae and a temporary change in sensation in the skin area of the incision,[11,18] which are obvious because of the surgical opening of the skin and superficial gland area. As mentioned before, development of sialoceles or fistula has not yet been observed by the authors and is not reported in the literature. The often-mentioned potential risk of facial nerve damage is based on the lack knowledge of anatomic and surgical skills as this nerve, as also mentioned before, is 1.5 to 2.0 cm below the surface of the gland. The only reported complications are a temporary change in sensation in the skin area of the incision. No permanent complications are, however, documented in the literature.[11,18,26] The level of postoperative pain accompanying a parotid gland biopsy is comparable with a lip biopsy.[11]

SUITABILITY OF SALIVARY GLAND BIOPSIES
Diagnostic

As mentioned before, a labial salivary gland biopsy is considered as positive for SS when focal lymphocytic sialadenitis with a focus score of 1 or greater per 4 mm^2 glandular tissue is present (see **Fig. 3**). However, for proper interpretation of the biopsy specimens broad experience is needed as focal lymphocytic sialadenitis may occur in conjunction with other autoimmune diseases and even in healthy subjects, in particular in the elderly.[27] Typically for pSS, the lymphocytic foci have to be adjacent to normal-appearing mucous acini and contain no more than a minority proportion of plasma cells. Furthermore, at greater than a focus score of 10, foci are typically confluent; an arbitrary score of 12 is often applied for such biopsies.[13,14] Other difficulties that may interfere with the interpretation of the biopsies are features more usually associated with nonspecific chronic sialadenitis, such as acinar atrophy, interstitial fibrosis, and duct dilatation. These features are relatively common and increase with age and may also coexist with pSS-related focal lymphocytic sialadenitis.[10,28] Replacement of glandular tissue with fibrotic tissue as a result of age and chronic salivary gland inflammation may lower the focus score and lead to a burnt-out appearance.[10,29] Moreover, it may be difficult to harvest a sufficient number of labial salivary glands in atrophic submucosa of patients with long-standing SS.[30]

In contrast to labial glands, parotid salivary biopsies allow the clinician to monitor disease progression and to assess the effect of an intervention treatment in SS. This assessment is feasible because parotid tissue can be harvested relative easily, repeated biopsies from the same parotid gland are possible, and the histopathologic results can be compared with other diagnostic results derived from the same gland (eg, secretory function, sialographic appearance, scintigraphy, ultrasound, computed tomography [CT], MRI).[31] Additionally, by performing parotid biopsies as a routine diagnostic procedure for SS, LELs and lymphomas located in the parotid gland can identified (see section on lymphoma).[18,32] So, the question remains as to what biopsy should be preferred for diagnostics and/or monitoring disease progression and treatment efficacy.

Disease Progression

There are only few studies that compared the diagnostic characteristics of major and minor salivary gland biopsies and even none that compared the ability of both biopsy types to monitor disease progression and treatment efficacy. Pijpe and colleagues[11] compared the diagnostic ability of labial and parotid salivary gland biopsies in diagnosing pSS as well as compared their morbidity. They showed that the diagnostic sensitivity and specificity were identical. Moreover, the presence of characteristic benign LELs in the parotid gland can aid the diagnosis of SS. The observation that LELs are commonly present in parotid biopsies and are virtually absent in labial salivary gland biopsies was earlier confirmed by Pennec and colleagues[33] and Carbone and colleagues.[34] The incidence of germinal centers in the major and minor salivary gland biopsies is comparable.[11] There is a need for larger studies comparing the diagnostic utility of labial and parotid salivary gland biopsies in the diagnostic work-up of SS emphasizing whether these procedures are exchangeable or that a specific biopsy type is preferred for a specific diagnostic issue regarding SS or SS-associated diseases.

Treatment Evaluation Purposes

EULAR has developed a disease activity index (EULAR Sjögren's Syndrome Disease Activity Index [ESSDAI]) and a patient-reported index (EULAR Sjögren's Syndrome Patient Reported Index [ESSPRI]) as validated outcome measures for SS.[35–38] Although the development is an important advantage, ESSDAI focuses on systemic disease features and is so less relevant to patients with predominantly glandular features. The ESSPRI addresses the symptomatic components of dryness, pain, and fatigue. Fatigue has an important impact on the quality of life but might be susceptible to placebo effects or the impact of concomitant disorders leading to important implications for sample size. Thus, as posed by Fisher and colleagues,[10] an objective biomarker of glandular inflammation would, therefore, be desirable; salivary gland biopsy has the added advantage that it may offer insights into the mechanism of action of a novel agent or, more importantly, reasons for failure in a negative study.

When comparing the potential application of labial and parotid salivary gland biopsies with regard to disease activity and progression, studies involving repeated labial salivary gland biopsies revealed that in patients presenting with sicca symptoms, a focus score of 1 or greater was associated with antibodies to Ro and La, rheumatoid factor, antinuclear antibody, and a lower unstimulated whole salivary flow rate.[4,39,40] It was also shown that a higher focus score is accompanied by a larger decrease in an unstimulated[41] and stimulated[42] whole salivary flow rate over time. Repeated labial salivary gland biopsies might have some value in assessing the effect of biologicals on the glandular level as labial salivary gland biopsies seems to be of added value in rating the efficacy of treatment with rituximab,[7] abatacept,[8] or belimumab.[9] It has to be mentioned, however, that the same labial salivary glands are not examined as a function of time but a new sample of glands collected from the same patient bringing the hazard of the reproducibility of, for example, a focus score in repeated sections from even the same labial salivary glands into mind.[16] However, Kapsogeorgou and colleagues[43] showed that the infiltration grade and prevalence of the major infiltrating cell types (T and B cells, macrophages, dendritic cells, natural killer cells) remained largely unchanged during a median 55-month biopsy time interval follow-up (quartiles 42–81) indicating that the labial salivary gland histopathology is rather stable with time and probably does not readily reflect disease progression and/or disease activity.

In contrast to labial salivary glands, repeated biopsies from the same parotid gland are possible, which is probably an important asset in studies assessing the efficacy of a treatment in patients with SS or monitoring disease progression. Another important advantage is that the histopathologic results can be compared with other diagnostic results derived from the same gland (secretory function, sialographic appearance, scintigraphy, ultrasound, CT, MRI). Moreover, as mentioned before, LELs are often observed in parotid gland tissue of patients with SS and rarely in labial salivary gland tissue. These LELs, a characteristic histologic feature of the major salivary glands in SS,[44] develop as a result of basal cell hyperplasia forming a multilayered epithelium. Between these reactive ductal epithelial cells, lymphocytes are present.[44]

Although features of labial salivary gland pathology have been associated with a variety of serologic, clinical, and imaging parameters, features of parotid salivary gland tissue are not yet associated with such parameters. However, currently several studies are underway assessing whether histopathologic features reflect changes in whole and glandular salivary flow, serum, and salivary gland ultrasonography. First results will become available shortly indicating whether disease progression and disease activity are indeed accompanied by characteristic features at the level of parotid gland histopathology. With regard to parotid salivary gland tissue as a monitor of treatment efficacy, more progress has been made. Pijpe and colleagues[31] showed in an open-label trial that sequential parotid biopsy specimens obtained from patients with pSS before and after rituximab treatment demonstrated histopathologic evidence of reduced glandular inflammation and redifferentiation of lymphoepithelial duct lesions to regular striated ducts as a putative morphologic correlate of increased parotid flow and normalization of the salivary sodium content. Next, Delli and colleagues[45] assessed the prognostic value of parotid gland immunopathology with regard to responsiveness of patients with pSS to rituximab treatment in a randomized placebo-controlled study. These investigators found a significant reduction in the number of CD20+ B cells per square millimeter of parenchyma, whereas no reduction was observed in placebo-treated patients. Furthermore, the relative number and severity of LELs and germinal centers significantly reduced after rituximab treatment. Moreover, when comparing the baseline characteristics of clinical responders with nonresponders to rituximab treatment, the number of CD20+ B cells per square millimeter of parenchyma was significantly higher in responders, which might predict the responsiveness of patients with pSS to rituximab treatment. In addition, an open-label study with abatacept[46] showed that treatment did not affect the focus score, area of lymphocytic infiltrate, and number of LELs infiltrating B and T cells. However, abatacept reduced the presence of germinal centers (GC), which was associated with an improvement in the glandular domain (reduction in swelling) of the ESSDAI. Thus, abatacept seems to inhibit local T-cell dependent B-cell activation in parotid gland tissue of patients with pSS as witnessed by the decline in GC per square millimeter after treatment. Furthermore, the presence of GC at baseline predicts response in ESSDAI glandular domain after abatacept treatment. These observations have to be confirmed in a placebo-controlled study, a study that is currently in progress.

SALIVARY GLAND BIOPSIES AND LYMPHOMAS

Five percent to 10% of patients with SS develop malignant B-cell lymphoma,[47–49] 48% to 75% of which are of the mucosa-associated lymphoid tissue (MALT)–type. These MALT B-cell lymphomas are most frequently located in the parotid gland.[50–52] Theander and colleagues[6] suggested that the presence of GC-like structures in pSS diagnostic labial salivary biopsies is highly predictive and an easy-to-obtain marker for non-Hodgkin lymphoma development. They even posed that presence of these GC-like structures allows for risk stratification of patients and the possibility to initiate preventive B-cell–directed therapy. Later on, however, Johnsen and colleagues[53] were unable to detect a clear association between cellular infiltrates, B-cell clonality, and lymphoma development in labial salivary gland biopsies. The authors' recent data indicate that presence of germinal centers in diagnostic (labial) biopsies is not a risk factor for the development of MALT lymphoma in the parotid glands.[54] Because lymphomas in patients with pSS mainly develop in parotid glands, taking parotid gland biopsies may be a great asset in both diagnosing pSS-associated lymphomas as well as in titrating which therapy is needed.[32] Quintana and colleagues[55] and De Vita and colleagues[56] mentioned that LELs and reactive lymphoid follicles, features that are commonplace in parotid salivary gland pathology of patients with pSS, indicate malignant lymphoma and, thus, benign LELs must be discriminated from premalignant lesions. Haacke and colleagues[54] looked with more detail into salivary gland biopsies of patients with pSS with regard to LELs and observed that FcRL4+ B cells are in close association with LELs and that these FcRL4+ B cells are significantly increased when comparing the parotid gland with the labial gland. As MALT lymphomas, and a small subset of diffuse B-cell lymphomas, express FcRL4,[57] this observation might explain why lymphomas in patients with pSS commonly develop in parotid and not in minor salivary glands and, thus, favors taking a parotid and not a labial salivary gland biopsy in the diagnostic work-up of patients with SS, at least in patients with a suspect of lymphoma development.

SUMMARY

Early diagnosis and objective treatment evaluation of costly therapies based on biologicals are of high importance in SS. Unfortunately, so far there is not a single test capable of confirming the diagnosis of SS. A positive salivary gland biopsy is strong evidence, which in correlation with additional diagnostic tests can establish a definite conclusion. Parotid gland biopsy is a relatively simple technique with no permanent morbidity reported compared with a relative high morbidity rate of labial salivary gland biopsies due to the rather high hazard of permanent damage to the sensory nerve supply of the lower lip in the latter biopsies. Parotid biopsies are able to overcome most of these disadvantages.

REFERENCES

1. Vitali C, Bombardieri S, Jonsson R, et al. Classification criteria for Sjögren's syndrome: a revised version of the European criteria proposed by the American-European Consensus Group. Ann Rheum Dis 2002;61(6):554–8.
2. Shiboski SC, Shiboski CH, Criswell L, et al. American College of Rheumatology classification criteria for Sjögren's syndrome: a data-driven, expert consensus approach in the Sjögren's International Collaborative Clinical Alliance cohort. Arthritis Care Res (Hoboken) 2012;64(4):475–87.
3. Chisholm DM, Mason DK. Labial salivary gland biopsy in Sjögren's disease. J Clin Pathol 1968;21(5):656–60.
4. Daniels TE, Cox D, Shiboski CH, et al. Associations between salivary gland histopathologic diagnoses and phenotypic features of Sjögren's syndrome among 1,726 registry participants. Arthritis Rheum 2011;63(7):2021–30.
5. Shiboski C, Shiboski S. Proposed ACR-EULAR classification criteria for Sjögren's syndrome: development and validation. Scand J Immunol 2015;81(5):330.
6. Theander E, Vasaitis L, Baecklund E, et al. Lymphoid organisation in labial salivary gland biopsies is a possible predictor for the development of malignant lymphoma in primary Sjögren's syndrome. Ann Rheum Dis 2011;70(8):1363–8.
7. Carubbi F, Cipriani P, Marrelli A, et al. Efficacy and safety of rituximab treatment in early primary Sjögren's syndrome: a prospective, multi-center, follow-up study. Arthritis Res Ther 2013;15(5):R172.
8. Adler S, Korner M, Forger F, et al. Evaluation of histologic, serologic, and clinical changes in response to abatacept treatment of primary Sjögren's syndrome: a pilot study. Arthritis Care Res (Hoboken) 2013;65(11):1862–8.
9. De Vita S, Quartuccio L, Seror R, et al. Efficacy and safety of belimumab given for 12 months in primary Sjögren's syndrome: the BELISS open-label phase II study. Rheumatology (Oxford) 2015;54(12):2249–56.
10. Fisher BA, Brown RM, Bowman SJ, et al. A review of salivary gland histopathology in primary Sjögren's syndrome with a focus on its potential as a clinical trials biomarker. Ann Rheum Dis 2015;74(9):1645–50.
11. Pijpe J, Kalk WW, van der Wal JE, et al. Parotid gland biopsy compared with labial biopsy in the diagnosis of patients with primary Sjögren's syndrome. Rheumatology (Oxford) 2007;46(2):335–41.
12. Vissink A, Bootsma H, Kroese FG, et al. How to assess treatment efficacy in Sjögren's syndrome? Curr Opin Rheumatol 2012;24(3):281–9.
13. Greenspan JS, Daniels TE, Talal N, et al. The histopathology of Sjögren's syndrome in labial salivary gland biopsies. Oral Surg Oral Med Oral Pathol 1974;37(2):217–29.
14. Daniels TE. Labial salivary gland biopsy in Sjögren's syndrome. Assessment as a diagnostic criterion in 362 suspected cases. Arthritis Rheum 1984;27(2):147–56.
15. Labial Salivary Glands Biopsy Histopathology SOP for SICCA Research Groups. 2005. Available at: https://sicca-online.ucsf.edu/documents/LSG_bx_Grading_SOP.pdf.
16. Al-Hashimi I, Wright JM, Cooley CA, et al. Reproducibility of biopsy grade in Sjögren's syndrome. J Oral Pathol Med 2001;30(7):408–12.
17. Friedman H, Kilmar V, Galletta VP, et al. Lip biopsy in connective tissue diseases. A review and study of seventy cases. Oral Surg Oral Med Oral Pathol 1979;47(3):256–62.

18. Marx RE, Hartman KS, Rethman KV. A prospective study comparing incisional labial to incisional parotid biopsies in the detection and confirmation of sarcoidosis, Sjögren's disease, sialosis and lymphoma. J Rheumatol 1988;15(4):621–9.
19. Delgado WA, Mosqueda A. A highly sensitive method for diagnosis of secondary amyloidosis by labial salivary gland biopsy. J Oral Pathol Med 1989;18(5):310–4.
20. Mahlstedt K, Ussmuller J, Donath K. Value of minor salivary gland biopsy in diagnosing Sjögren's syndrome. J Otolaryngol 2002;31(5):299–303.
21. Berquin K, Mahy P, Weynand B, et al. Accessory or sublingual salivary gland biopsy to assess systemic disease: a comparative retrospective study. Eur Arch Otorhinolaryngol 2006;263(3):233–6.
22. Caporali R, Bonacci E, Epis O, et al. Comment on: parotid gland biopsy compared with labial biopsy in the diagnosis of patients with primary Sjögren's syndrome. Rheumatology (Oxford) 2007;46(10):1625 [author reply: 1625–6].
23. Teppo H, Revonta M. A follow-up study of minimally invasive lip biopsy in the diagnosis of Sjögren's syndrome. Clin Rheumatol 2007;26(7):1099–103.
24. Richards A, Mutlu S, Scully C, et al. Complications associated with labial salivary gland biopsy in the investigation of connective tissue disorders. Ann Rheum Dis 1992;51(8):996–7.
25. Kraaijenhagen HA. Letter: technique for parotid biopsy. J Oral Surg 1975;33(5):328.
26. Delli K, Vissink A, Spijkervet FK. Salivary gland biopsy for Sjögren's syndrome. Oral Maxillofac Surg Clin North Am 2014;26(1):23–33.
27. Radfar L, Kleiner DE, Fox PC, et al. Prevalence and clinical significance of lymphocytic foci in minor salivary glands of healthy volunteers. Arthritis Rheum 2002;47(5):520–4.
28. Scott J. Qualitative and quantitative observations on the histology of human labial salivary glands obtained post mortem. J Biol Buccale 1980;8(3):187–200.
29. Bookman AA, Shen H, Cook RJ, et al. Whole stimulated salivary flow: correlation with the pathology of inflammation and damage in minor salivary gland biopsy specimens from patients with primary Sjögren's syndrome but not patients with sicca. Arthritis Rheum 2011;63(7):2014–20.
30. Vitali C, Tavoni A, Simi U, et al. Parotid sialography and minor salivary gland biopsy in the diagnosis of Sjögren's syndrome. A comparative study of 84 patients. J Rheumatol 1988;15(2):262–7.
31. Pijpe J, Meijer JM, Bootsma H, et al. Clinical and histologic evidence of salivary gland restoration supports the efficacy of rituximab treatment in Sjögren's syndrome. Arthritis Rheum 2009;60(11):3251–6.
32. Pollard RP, Pijpe J, Bootsma H, et al. Treatment of mucosa-associated lymphoid tissue lymphoma in Sjögren's syndrome: a retrospective clinical study. J Rheumatol 2011;38(10):2198–208.
33. Pennec YL, Leroy JP, Jouquan J, et al. Comparison of labial and sublingual salivary gland biopsies in the diagnosis of Sjögren's syndrome. Ann Rheum Dis 1990;49(1):37–9.
34. Carbone A, Gloghini A, Ferlito A. Pathological features of lymphoid proliferations of the salivary glands: lymphoepithelial sialadenitis versus low-grade B-cell lymphoma of the malt type. Ann Otol Rhinol Laryngol 2000;109(12 Pt 1):1170–5.
35. Seror R, Ravaud P, Bowman SJ, et al. EULAR Sjögren's syndrome disease activity index: development of a consensus systemic disease activity index for primary Sjögren's syndrome. Ann Rheum Dis 2010;69(6):1103–9.
36. Seror R, Ravaud P, Mariette X, et al. EULAR Sjögren's Syndrome Patient Reported Index (ESSPRI): development of a consensus patient index for primary Sjögren's syndrome. Ann Rheum Dis 2011;70(6):968–72.

37. Seror R, Bootsma H, Saraux A, et al. Defining disease activity states and clinically meaningful improvement in primary Sjögren's syndrome with EULAR primary Sjögren's syndrome disease activity (ESSDAI) and patient-reported indexes (ESSPRI). Ann Rheum Dis 2016;75:382–9.

38. Seror R, Theander E, Brun JG, et al. Validation of EULAR primary Sjögren's syndrome disease activity (ESSDAI) and patient indexes (ESSPRI). Ann Rheum Dis 2015;74(5):859–66.

39. Dinerman H, Goldenberg DL, Felson DT. A prospective evaluation of 118 patients with the fibromyalgia syndrome: prevalence of Raynaud's phenomenon, sicca symptoms, ANA, low complement, and Ig deposition at the dermal-epidermal junction. J Rheumatol 1986;13(2):368–73.

40. Rhodus NL, Fricton J, Carlson P, et al. Oral symptoms associated with fibromyalgia syndrome. J Rheumatol 2003;30(8):1841–5.

41. Haldorsen K, Moen K, Jacobsen H, et al. Exocrine function in primary Sjögren syndrome: natural course and prognostic factors. Ann Rheum Dis 2008;67(7): 949–54.

42. Jonsson R, Kroneld U, Backman K, et al. Progression of sialadenitis in Sjögren's syndrome. Br J Rheumatol 1993;32(7):578–81.

43. Kapsogeorgou EK, Christodoulou MI, Panagiotakos DB, et al. Minor salivary gland inflammatory lesions in Sjögren syndrome: do they evolve? J Rheumatol 2013;40(9):1566–71.

44. Ihrler S, Zietz C, Sendelhofert A, et al. Lymphoepithelial duct lesions in Sjögren-type sialadenitis. Virchows Arch 1999;434(4):315–23.

45. Delli K, Haacke EA, Pollard RP, et al. Baseline characteristics of parotid gland histopatholology predict responsiveness of patients with primary Sjögren's syndrome to rituximab treatment. Scand J Immunol 2015;81(5):329–450.

46. Haacke EA, van der Vegt B, Meiners PM, et al. Germinal centers disappear in parotid gland tissue after treatment of primary Sjögren's syndrome with abatacept. Scand J Immunol 2015;81(5):437–8.

47. Sutcliffe N, Inanc M, Speight P, et al. Predictors of lymphoma development in primary Sjögren's syndrome. Semin Arthritis Rheum 1998;28(2):80–7.

48. Theander E, Henriksson G, Ljungberg O, et al. Lymphoma and other malignancies in primary Sjögren's syndrome: a cohort study on cancer incidence and lymphoma predictors. Ann Rheum Dis 2006;65(6):796–803.

49. Nocturne G, Mariette X. Sjögren syndrome-associated lymphomas: an update on pathogenesis and management. Br J Haematol 2015;168(3):317–27.

50. Kassan SS, Thomas TL, Moutsopoulos HM, et al. Increased risk of lymphoma in sicca syndrome. Ann Intern Med 1978;89(6):888–92.

51. Tzioufas AG, Boumba DS, Skopouli FN, et al. Mixed monoclonal cryoglobulinemia and monoclonal rheumatoid factor cross-reactive idiotypes as predictive factors for the development of lymphoma in primary Sjögren's syndrome. Arthritis Rheum 1996;39(5):767–72.

52. Voulgarelis M, Dafni UG, Isenberg DA, et al. Malignant lymphoma in primary Sjögren's syndrome: a multicenter, retrospective, clinical study by the European Concerted Action on Sjögren's Syndrome. Arthritis Rheum 1999;42(8):1765–72.

53. Johnsen SJ, Berget E, Jonsson MV, et al. Evaluation of germinal center-like structures and B cell clonality in patients with primary Sjögren syndrome with and without lymphoma. J Rheumatol 2014;41(11):2214–22.

54. Haacke EA, Kluin PM, Vissink A, et al. Salivary gland FcRL4(+) B-cells are a potential source of progenitor cells for MALT lymphoma in primary Sjögren's syndrome. Scand J Immunol 2015;81(5):380–1.

55. Quintana PG, Kapadia SB, Bahler DW, et al. Salivary gland lymphoid infiltrates associated with lymphoepithelial lesions: a clinicopathologic, immunophenotypic, and genotypic study. Hum Pathol 1997;28(7):850–61.

56. De Vita S, De Marchi G, Sacco S, et al. Preliminary classification of nonmalignant B cell proliferation in Sjögren's syndrome: perspectives on pathobiology and treatment based on an integrated clinico-pathologic and molecular study approach. Blood Cells Mol Dis 2001;27(4):757–66.

57. Falini B, Agostinelli C, Bigerna B, et al. IRTA1 is selectively expressed in nodal and extranodal marginal zone lymphomas. Histopathology 2012;61(5):930–41.

58. Guevara-Gutierrez E, Tlacuilo-Parra A, Minjares-Padilla LM. Minor salivary gland punch biopsy for evaluation of Sjögren's syndrome. J Clin Rheumatol 2001;7(6): 401–2.

59. Gorson KC, Ropper AH. Positive salivary gland biopsy, Sjögren syndrome, and neuropathy: clinical implications. Muscle Nerve 2003;28(5):553–60.

60. McGuirt WF Jr, Whang C, Moreland W. The role of parotid biopsy in the diagnosis of pediatric Sjögren syndrome. Arch Otolaryngol Head Neck Surg 2002;128(11): 1279–81.

61. Baurmash H. Parotid biopsy technique. J Oral Maxillofac Surg 2005;63(10): 1556–7.

62. Adam P, Haroun A, Billet J, et al. Biopsy of the salivary glands. The importance and technic of biopsy of the sublingual gland on its anterio-lateral side. Rev Stomatol Chir Maxillofac 1992;93(5):337–40.

Major Salivary Gland Ultrasonography in the Diagnosis of Sjögren's Syndrome

A Place in the Diagnostic Criteria?

Malin V. Jonsson, DMD, PhD[a,b,*], Chiara Baldini, MD, PhD[c]

KEYWORDS

- Imaging • Major salivary gland • Ultrasonography • Ultrasound
- Sjögren's syndrome

KEY POINTS

- Salivary gland ultrasonography (SG-US) represents a useful imaging method for detecting structural abnormalities in the major SGs in patients with Sjögren syndrome (SS).
- SG-US may serve as a first-line imaging tool in the diagnosis of primary SS (pSS) and should be included in the diagnostic criteria.
- Studies are needed to demonstrate the reliability of the US technique and its sensitivity to change in the management of patients with pSS.

INTRODUCTION

Primary Sjögren syndrome (pSS) is an autoimmune chronic inflammatory disease predominantly affecting the salivary and lacrimal glands with progressive focal mono-nuclear cell infiltration (**Fig. 1**), loss of salivary gland (SG) acinar epithelial tissue, and degenerative changes, such as fibrosis,[1] and giving rise to clinical symptoms, such as oral and ocular dryness (xerostomia and keratoconjunctivitis sicca, respectively). The disease manifestations vary greatly, from very mild symptoms of dryness, to severe extraglandular manifestations of the lung, kidney, liver, neurological, and hemato-logical system.[2] Fatigue is a common feature of pSS,[3] but by far the most severe

Disclosures: No disclosures.
[a] Section for Oral and Maxillofacial Radiology, Department of Clinical Dentistry, Faculty of Medicine and Dentistry, University of Bergen, Årstadveien 19, Bergen N-5009, Norway; [b] Broegelmann Research Laboratory, Department of Clinical Medicine, Faculty of Medicine and Dentistry, University of Bergen, Bergen, Norway; [c] Rheumatology Unit, University of Pisa, Roma 67, 56126 Pisa, Italy
* Corresponding author. Section for Oral and Maxillofacial Radiology, Department of Clinical Dentistry, Årstadveien 19, Bergen N-5009, Norway.
E-mail address: malin.jonsson@uib.no

Rheum Dis Clin N Am 42 (2016) 501–517
http://dx.doi.org/10.1016/j.rdc.2016.03.008
0889-857X/16/$ – see front matter © 2016 Elsevier Inc. All rights reserved.
rheumatic.theclinics.com

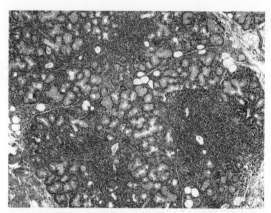

Fig. 1. Minor salivary gland biopsy with 3 distinct focal mononuclear cell infiltrates, located around epithelial ducts (periductal) and surrounded by otherwise normal-appearing acinar epithelial cells.

complication of pSS is lymphoma,[4] most commonly non-Hodgkin lymphoma occurring in 4% to 5% of patients with pSS,[5] with an estimated 16 times increased risk in comparison with the background population.[6]

The diagnosis of pSS is based on 6 items according to the American-European consensus group (AECG) classification criteria for pSS of 2002.[7] According to these criteria, the assessment of SG involvement in SS is based on focal mononuclear cell infiltrates in the minor SGs (see **Fig. 1**), by measures of unstimulated salivary secretion (sialometry) and/or by the detection of morphologic and functional abnormalities of the glands by scintigraphy or sialography, as well as subjective symptoms of oral dryness (xerostomia). In 2012, the American College of Rheumatology (ACR) presented an alternate version of the criteria,[8] based on the Sjögren's International Collaborative Clinical Alliance(SICCA) cohort, comprising a group of clinical and laboratory investigators, a biorepository, and a data registry. Whereas the AECG 2002 criteria[7] consist of both subjective symptoms, such as dryness of the mouth and eyes, and objective findings of reduced saliva and tear production, the ACR 2012 criteria[8] has weighted the autoimmune and eye components, practically excluding the oral and salivary components, with an exception for minor SG biopsy and sialometry.

A novel set of classification criteria for SS was recently presented,[9,10] intending to give researchers a single set of consensus measures for the classification of SS, and aiming to replace both the provisional 2012 ACR criteria[8] and the 2002 AECG criteria.[7] The novel criteria are based on 5 objective tests or items, resulting in a total score ≥ 4, derived from the sum of the weights assigned to each positive test/item. Focus score (FS) ≥ 1 and positive anti-Ro/SSA serology are proposed to have the highest weighting (3 for each positive test), whereas Ocular Staining Score (OSS) ≥ 5 on at least 1 eye, Schirmer I-test ≤ 5 mm/5 minutes on at least 1 eye, and unstimulated whole salivary flow rate ≤ 0.1 mL/min, will have a weighting of 1 for each positive test. The involvement of SGs is documented by unstimulated sialometry and/or by the minor SG biopsy.

Keeping in mind, classification criteria were essentially developed to classify clinical trial participants, and not for diagnostic purposes. Hence, the diagnostic armamentarium for the SG component in pSS may still count on a broad spectrum of diagnostic tools including sialography (**Fig. 2**) and scintigraphy. In this scenario, a growing

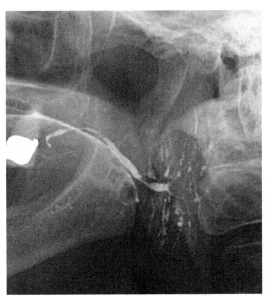

Fig. 2. Sialography of the left parotid gland, showing evenly distributed contrast medium in the glandular structures, with thin, delicate ducts and several areas of acinar filling (sialectasis). (*Courtesy of* Skaale SG, MD, University of Bergen, Bergen, Norway.)

interest has arisen for major SG ultrasonography (SG-US), which has appeared as a valuable, noninvasive, reproducible tool for the diagnosis of SS.[11] SG-US has also been applied to assess SG involvement in secondary Sjögren syndrome (sSS), another condition for which the novel ACR/AECG criteria have not been validated.[12–14]

The aim of this review was to go through recent literature of SG-US in SS, and to assess its diagnostic and prognostic value in clinical practice as well as in clinical trials.

MODALITIES FOR SALIVARY GLAND IMAGING

Several imaging modalities have been investigated for evaluation of the SG involvement in pSS,[15] with chronic inflammatory changes seemingly occurring in the submandibular glands before the parotid glands.[16] In sialography (see **Fig. 2**), a contrast medium commonly containing iodine is administered to the glandular tissue by a retrograde injection, providing a good illustration of the ductal structures, and been considered the gold standard for showing ductal inflammatory changes.[17,18] However, due to the partly invasive nature of sialography, it is contraindicated in patients with severe glandular dysfunction, and has in part been replaced by magnetic resonance (MR)-sialography.[19] Nuclear medicine, sialoscintigraphy, provides a quantitative measure of the SG function by imaging the uptake and excretion of a radioactive tracer (99mTc-sodium pertechnetate). In cases in which the labial SG biopsy is insufficient or not possible to perform, there is a potential diagnostic role for sialographic and scintigraphic examination[15] with diffuse sialectasis by parotid sialography (see **Fig. 2**), or salivary scintigraphy showing delayed uptake, reduced concentration, and/or delayed excretion of tracer.[7]

Ultrasonography and Sialography

Sonographic diagnostic criteria for SS were retrospectively investigated in a cohort of patients with previously suspected SS.[20] Ultrasonographic features, such as multiple hypoechoic areas, multiple hyperechoic lines or spots, multiple hypoechoic areas surrounded with hyperechoic lines or spots, and obscuration of the gland configuration were applied. Using logistic regression analysis, valuable sonographic findings were extracted, and sonographic images of a new group of patients investigated prospectively. Experienced observers were able to differentiate patients with SS from negative controls, and findings correlated well with sialographic grading, suggesting that SG-US can be substituted for sialography in screening for SS.

Using indices obtained by texture analyses of US parotid gland images of patients with a clinical suspicion of pSS (n = 132), patients fulfilling the revised Japanese criteria for SS[21] were identified (n = 91) and disease severity assessed.[22] Major SG-US findings (Hurst index) correlated with the degree of destruction of the parotid gland as determined by sialography, whereas the Hurst coefficient of the punctate stage, however, was almost similar to that of the normal stage.

The same group performed quantitative analyses (particle analysis, fractional Brownian motion [fBM] model analysis, 2-dimensional [2-D] fractal analysis) on US images of the parotid SG, and then evaluated whether the obtained indices correlated with the sialographic stage of Rubin-Holt in patients (n = 192) with a clinical suspicion of SS due to sicca symptoms, serologic findings, or neurologic symptoms.[23] Abnormal sialography findings were determined in a little less than half of the patient group. Indices of the parotid glands were entered into a logistic regression analysis to evaluate useful predictors for an abnormal sialographic stage. Significant differences were observed between the normal and abnormal groups in all 5 indices, and abnormal sialographic findings detected by quantitative analysis indicate a potential clinical application.

Consecutive patients (n = 105) were investigated by both high-resolution SG-US and sialography of the parotid glands,[24] and results retrospectively compared with the final diagnosis based on the AECG criteria.[7] Diagnosis of SS was confirmed in 45 patients; pSS (n = 36) and sSS (n = 9), and excluded in 15 subjects. The remaining subjects were excluded from the study due to incomplete records. A decreased and heterogeneous honeycomb pattern of parotid gland ultrasonography was observed in patients with SS, whereas sialography demonstrated a punctate pattern of sialectasis. Sensitivity, specificity, and accuracy for ultrasonography were 84.44%, 73.0%, and 81.6%, respectively, and 77.77%, 86.66%, and 80.0%, respectively, for conventional sialography. Interestingly, the diagnostic difference between the 2 investigations approached significance (P = .074), but by combining both imaging modalities, sensitivity increased to 91% with 60% specificity and 83.3% accuracy. Although not being able to separate pSS and sSS, high-resolution US was found more sensitive than sialography, and supplementing US with sialography increased accuracy.

Ultrasonography of the parotid and submandibular glands was investigated as an alternative to parotid sialography[25] in patients suspected of SS (n = 360). Patients (n = 188) fulfilled the AECG criteria for pSS (n = 134) and sSS (n = 54), or were classified as non-SS (n = 172). Glands were considered positive for SS if they exhibited peripheral sialectatic changes on sialography and/or hypoechoic areas, echogenic streaks and/or irregular gland margins on SG-US. Images were blindly rated as SS-positive or SS-negative. Average kappa values for the interobserver agreement were 0.81, 0.80, and 0.82 for sialography, parotid, and submandibular US, respectively, thus indicating very good or good agreement. Kappa value for intermodality agreement between sialography and parotid US was 0.81 and between sialography and submandibular US was 0.76, indicating very good and good agreement, respectively. Hence, the diagnostic ability of parotid US was lower than for sialography, but interestingly the diagnostic ability of submandibular US was comparable to that of sialography, prevailing submandibular US as a promising practical alternative to sialography in the classification of SS.

The diagnostic performance of sialography and SG-US for SS was also addressed in a meta-analysis.[26] Findings from 6 existing studies including patients (n = 488) and controls (n = 447) from 2 European and 4 Asian studies indicated that the diagnostic accuracy of SG-US is comparable with sialography in patients with SS.

Ultrasonography and Sialoscintigraphy

Salivary gland US was compared with sialoscintigraphy in the evaluation of SG function in patients diagnosed with SS.[27] In 2 patients with discordant results between sialoscintigraphy and SG-US, a labial biopsy was performed in addition. Abnormal sialoscintigrams were observed in 1 or more of the glands in 17 of 20 patients, and results confirmed by SG-US (n = 15) and labial minor SG biopsy (n = 2). In the remaining 3 patients with SS, both tests showed normal results. The study concluded that parotid and submandibular gland function was better identified by sialoscintigrams as compared with SG-US, as a more sensitive method and better indicating the stage of SS.[27]

US of the parotid and submandibular glands was compared to contrast sialography and scintigraphy[28] in patients fulfilling AECG criteria for pSS[7] (n = 77) and age-matched and sex-matched individuals with sicca symptoms (n = 79). SG-US imaging findings were graded using a score 0 to 16 based on the sum of scores for the parotid and submandibular glands. Sialographic and scintigraphic patterns were classified in 4 different stages. Pathologic SG-US findings were observed in 66 of 77 patients, abnormal sialographic findings in 59 of 77 patients, and abnormal scintigraphic findings in 58 of 77 patients, indicating SG-US as the best screening method, followed by sialography and SG scintigraphy. Adjusting the cutoff score greater than 6 SG-US provided a better ratio of sensitivity (75.3%) to specificity (83.5%), with a likelihood ratio of 4.58, whereas a threshold greater than 8.0 gained test specificity at the cost of sensitivity, with sensitivity 54.5%, specificity 97.5%, and likelihood ratio 21.5.

An SG-US scoring system of the parotid and submandibular glands (scale 0–48) was investigated as a less-invasive alternative to scintigraphy and minor SG biopsy[29] in patients with suspected SS (n = 135), establishing pSS diagnosis (n = 128) according to the AECG criteria.[7] Patients not fulfilling criteria for pSS according to the AECG criteria constituted the control group (n = 28). Patients' total scintigraphic score (0–12 scale) was determined and the minor SG histopathological changes graded. Major SG-US changes were detected in 98 of 107 patients with SS and in 14 of 28 controls, and SG-US arose as the best diagnostic test, followed by scintigraphy. Setting the SG-US cutoff score at 19 resulted in the best ratio of specificity (90.8%) to sensitivity (87.1%), whereas the scintigraphic cutoff score at 6 resulted in specificity of 86.1% and sensitivity of 67.1%. Among the 70 patients with SG-US score of 19 or higher, a scintigraphic score greater than 6 was recorded in 54 (77.1%) of 70 and positive biopsy findings in 62 (88.5%) of 70 patients.

In a cohort of patients (n = 190), the same group evaluated the diagnostic accuracy of SG-US as an alternative to scintigraphy in the AECG criteria,[7] by testing 3 different sets of 5 diagnostic criteria.[30] Each set combined ocular symptoms, oral symptoms, Schirmer I-test, and anti-Ro/SSA, with SG-US, sialoscintigraphy, or minor SG biopsy. SG-US score was positive in 129 (92%), sialoscintigraphy in 123 (88%), and biopsy in 93 (66%) of 140 patients with pSS. Among the patients with pSS (n = 140), 88 (63%) patients fulfilled the criteria with a positive SG-US, 85 (61%) patients with a positive sialoscintigraphy, and 71 (51%) patients with a positive minor SG biopsy. The non-pSS subjects (n = 50) did not fulfill any of the sets of criteria. Diagnostic accuracy was high for the SG-US, followed by the sialoscintigraphy and the minor SG biopsy.

Taking a different approach, the diagnostic value of SG scintigraphy was investigated in patients (n = 47) with diseases affecting the SGs.[31] All patients were investigated with SG scintigraphy. Patients with chronic obstructive parotitis (n = 25) also underwent SG-US, sialography, and sialoendoscopy; patients with sialolithiasis (n = 12) also underwent SG-US and computed tomography; and patients with SS (n = 10) also underwent SG-US and sialography. Patients with chronic obstructive parotitis showed reduced excretion of tracer by the affected glands, whereas uptake was nearly normal. The patients with sialolithiasis showed reduced excretion by the affected glands, and decreased uptake in 5 patients. In patients with SS, a decrease in both excretion and uptake by the 4 glands was shown.

NOVEL PERSPECTIVES
Gray Scale and Color/Power Doppler

Color Doppler, taking into use the principle that the sound pitch increases as the sound moves towards the listener, and decreases as it moves away, enables the imaging of blood flow and allows the clinician to see organ functioning in real time. With the addition of color it is possible to show the direction and rate of blood flow. With power Doppler US, the power in the Doppler signal is encoded in color, a fundamentally different parameter, from the mean frequency shift. The frequency is determined by the velocity of the red blood cells, whereas the power depends on the amount of blood present. Providing an image of a different property of blood flow, power Doppler has shown several key advantages over color Doppler, including higher sensitivity to flow, better edge definition, and depiction of continuity of flow. The combination of gray-scale SG-US and the color/power Doppler technique is suggested to provide more details with regard to soft tissue blood perfusion, and may be of value for narrowing in the number of differential diagnoses.[32]

In pSS, SG-US with color Doppler has been used to evaluate the major SG treatment response in following rituximab treatment.[33] Using B-mode US features, such as parenchymal homogeneity and gland size, and Doppler waveform analysis of the transverse facial artery of parotid glands, patients (n = 16) fulfilling the AECG criteria for pSS[7] were investigated and compared with controls (n = 9). The same US parameters were recorded before and after 12 weeks of intravenous rituximab therapy, and untreated patients had significant SG-US abnormalities in the SG structure and parotid size. Doppler waveform analysis showed significant differences before, but not after, lemon stimulation between untreated patients and controls. Following rituximab treatment, both the parotid and submandibular glands showed significant reduction in size compared with baseline. Doppler resistive indices after lemon stimulation were significantly increased after rituximab treatment.[33]

In a more recent study, the same group investigated SG echostructure and vascularization after rituximab treatment in patients with pSS (n = 28) included in the multicenter, randomized, double-blind, placebo-controlled trial Tolerance and Efficacy of Rituximab in Primary Sjögren's Syndrome (TEARS).[34] Patients with pSS[7] were examined with SG-US before the first placebo (n = 14) or rituximab infusion (n = 14), and 6 months after. US of the parotid and submandibular glands was performed and parameters echostructure (score 0–4), size of each gland, and vascularization based on the resistive index of the transverse facial artery of the parotid gland before and after lemon juice stimulation. At baseline 5 of 28 patients (3 in the placebo group and 2 in the rituximab group) had bilateral parotid gland enlargement. Parotid parenchyma echostructure improved in 50% of the rituximab-treated patients compared with 7% of the placebo-treated patients ($P = .03$). Submandibular gland echostructure also improved in a larger proportion of rituximab-treated patients, although not significantly. Size of the glands and resistive index remained unchanged.[34]

Parotid gland vascularity also has been studied as a diagnostic tool to improve the ultrasonographic diagnosis of SS.[35] Sonographic images of 72 cases of suspected SS, including 43 patients fulfilling the revised Japanese criteria for SS,[21] were analyzed retrospectively for the abnormal vascularity in the parotid gland parenchyma. Vascularity and the results of sialographic, serologic, and histopathologic examinations also were analyzed. The diagnostic accuracy of B-mode only was compared with B-mode plus Doppler-mode. Patients with SS showed significantly higher vascularity; and as the grade of vascularity increased, the rate of non-SS individuals decreased. The initial stage and cavitary-destructive stages showed the highest mean vascular score. Sensitivity and accuracy of B-mode were markedly increased with vascular information, and improving sonographic diagnosis for SS.

Contrast-Enhanced Ultrasonography

In contrast-enhanced SG-US, a contrast medium such as a small air bubble or a more complex structure, influencing the way the sound waves are reflected from interfaces between substances, is used. The technique was applied to distinguish SS from non-SS in a group of patients with sicca syndrome.[36] Patients with sicca syndrome were classified according to the AECG criteria,[7] and fulfilled criteria for pSS (n = 23) and sSS (n = 17). Patients not fulfilling criteria served as controls (n = 20). Contrast-enhanced US imaging of the parotid SGs was performed using a second-generation contrast agent with analysis of time-intensity curves at rest and during salivary stimulation. Sialoscintigraphy and minor labial SG biopsy also were performed. SG-US enhancement values were significantly lower in patients with pSS/sSS compared with individuals without SS, both at rest and during stimulation. Interestingly, in patients with pSS, enhancement values during stimulation were significantly lower compared with sSS. Contrast-enhanced SG-US imaging allowed discrimination of SS from non-SS sicca controls with 87.5% sensitivity, 85% specificity, and 86.7% accuracy, and pSS from sSS with 78.2% sensitivity, 70.5% specificity, and 75.0% accuracy.

Sonoelastography

The US technique real-time sonoelastography (RTS) is commonly used to investigate the elasticity of soft tissues, based on the principle that tissue compression produces strain (displacement) within the tissue that is less pronounced in harder compared with softer tissues.[37] The use of RTS of the major SGs was prospectively investigated for the assessment of glandular damage and diagnosis of pSS.[38] The cohort contained patients with pSS (n = 45) according to the AECG criteria,[7] individuals with sicca complaints (n = 24), and healthy controls (n = 11). Questionnaires, Saxon and Schirmer I-tests, and routine blood tests were carried out in all patients. All patients were investigated with B-mode SG-US and RTS of the parotid and submandibular glands, with abnormal findings graded 0 to 48 and 0 to 16, respectively. Sialoscintigraphy was performed with scores 0 to 12. Patients with pSS had higher B-mode scores compared with the sicca controls. In cases with an inconclusive B-mode SG-US, RTS cutoff score ≥6 provided a sensitive (66.7%) and specific (85.7%) classification of patients and sicca controls. In multivariate regression analysis, impaired SG function was reflected by RTS but not B-mode SG-US, but SG-US results were not related to any of the subjective dryness or discomfort measures. Sialoscintigraphy scores were associated with both B-mode SG-US and RTS results. Reproducibility of B-mode SG-US and RTS was good with intraclass correlation coefficients 0.93 and 0.93, respectively.[38]

SG elasticity also can be measured using Acoustic Radiation Force Impulse (ARFI) US, where local tissue displacement by a brief acoustic radiation induces the emission and propagation of shear waves, which are then digitally recorded. Shear wave velocity (SWV) is measured in meters per second and increases with tissue stiffness. SG-US with ARFI elastometry was performed in healthy controls (n = 15) and patients with pSS (n = 10).[39] Patients were classified according to the ACR criteria.[8] In the parotid glands, mean SWV was significantly higher in the pSS group than in the control group ($P = .001$), whereas mean SWV values for the submandibular glands were not significantly different between the patients and controls ($P = .892$).

Another recent study also evaluated SG stiffness in pSS using quantitative ARFI imaging, including Virtual Touch tissue quantification (VTQ) and Virtual Touch tissue imaging quantification (VTIQ).[40] VTQ was used to calculate the SWV, providing an objective numerical evaluation of the tissue stiffness, whereas VTIQ, a 2D shear wave imaging displaying a color-coded image, was used to enable the detection of SWV in multiple locations. Patients with pSS (n = 21) according to the AECG criteria[7] and healthy controls (n = 11) were included, and both parotid and submandibular glands were examined using VTQ and VTIQ. The parotid VTQ value was significantly higher in the pSS group than the control group ($P<.01$). Interestingly, VTIQ values for both the parotid and submandibular glands were significantly higher in the pSS group than in the control group ($P<.05$), and the VTQ and VTIQ results correlated for the parotid and submandibular glands.

DIAGNOSTIC APPLICATIONS AND PROGNOSTIC VALUE
Scoring Systems

In 1992, De Vita and colleagues[12] presented initial guidelines for US evaluation of SG abnormalities in SS. A series of different US abnormalities, including glandular size, echogenicity, and inhomogeneity, were investigated for their discriminant power for SS. The cohort consisted of 53 patients with either pSS (n = 27) or sSS (n = 26) classified according to the Copenhagen criteria for SS,[41] as well as controls (n = 90). The controls suffered from dry mouth and/or recurrent/persistent major SG swelling (n = 26), or were healthy, asymptomatic individuals (n = 64). When comparing patients with controls, the variables mild, evident, or gross inhomogeneous parenchymal patterns were selected by stepwise discriminant analysis. However, mild submandibular inhomogeneity did not prove useful for such discrimination. Based on these data, a simplified evaluation and standardized quantification of salivary involvement was proposed using an echographic score (0–6), assigning points to the degrees of glandular inhomogeneity. Score values above 0 showed a sensitivity of 88.8% in primary SS and of 53.8% in secondary SS, as well as specificity of 84.6% and of 92.2% with respect to either symptomatic or healthy controls.

Hocevar and colleagues[42] performed US of both parotid and submandibular glands in consecutive patients with suspected SS (n = 218), in addition to the regular diagnostic procedure following the AECG criteria.[7] The study comprised patients fulfilling criteria for SS (n = 68) and controls (n = 150) in whom SS was not confirmed. Several US parameters, including echogenicity, inhomogeneity, number of hypoechogenic areas, the hyperechogenic reflections, and clearness of the SG borders, were evaluated, and the 5 parameters summarized for all 4 major SGs. The final SG-US score ranged from 0 to 48. All 5 SG-US parameters were significantly associated with SS, and setting the SG-US score cutoff at 17 resulted in the best ratio of specificity (98.7%) to sensitivity (58.8%).

Reproducibility of the semiquantitative scoring system was determined in patients with SS (n = 28) according to the AECG criteria[7] and controls (n = 29).[43] The parotid and submandibular glands were independently evaluated by 2 blinded investigators assessing echogenicity, delineation of glandular borders, and sonographic structure, including homogeneity, hypoechoic areas, and hyperechoic foci. A high degree of interobserver agreement was determined regarding the final SG-US score (0.90) and the assessment of glandular homogeneity (0.90), echogenicity (0.88), and hypoechoic areas (0.88).

In 2013, Cornec and colleagues[14] performed SG-US in a prospective cohort of patients with suspected pSS (n = 158). Major SG-US cutoff ≥ 2 was able to distinguish patients with pSS (n = 78) from controls (n = 80) with a sensitivity of 62.8%, specificity of 95.0%, 92.5% positive predictive value, and 72.4% negative predictive value, compared with the AECG critera[7] and clinical assessment by a group of experts. Similarly, Baldini and colleagues[44] tested the accuracy of SG-US for the early detection of pSS and compared the diagnostic performance of SG-US with minor SG biopsy and unstimulated whole salivary flow rate in this context. The study included subjects with suspected pSS (n = 107) and symptom duration of ≤ 5 years, whereas 50 patients fulfilled criteria for pSS.[7] The SG-US cutoff ≥ 1 obtained a sensitivity of 66%, a specificity of 98%, a positive predictive value of 97%, and a negative predictive value of 73% for the diagnosis of pSS. The SG-US score also correlated with patients' minor SG focus score and unstimulated whole saliva.

Performance of SG-US was also explored for the diagnosis of sSS or pSS with respect to other systemic autoimmune disorders in a clinical rheumatology setting.[13] Wernicke and colleagues investigated consecutive patients with rheumatic diseases (n = 316), and found that evident parenchymal inhomogenicity in 2 or more major SGs allowed the differentiation between pSS (n = 57) and sSS (n = 33) according to the AECG criteria,[7] with a sensitivity of 63.1% and 63.6%, respectively. The specificity of the applied SG-US imaging approach in the cohort was 98.7%. Interestingly, the volume of submandibular glands was reduced by about 30% in patients with pSS and sSS compared with patients with sicca symptoms (n = 78) and asymptomatic controls (n = 148). Although reduced volumes of both submandibular glands in pSS and sSS had a specificity of 93% and a sensitivity of 48% at the cutoff point of 3.0 mL, the volume of the parotid glands did not differ between the groups of patients. Parenchymal inhomogeneity was strongly associated with anti-Ro/SSA and/or anti-La/SSB autoantibodies in patients with pSS.

Milic and colleagues[45] analyzed the SG-US performance in consecutive patients with rheumatic diseases (n = 209). Patients were classified according to the AECG criteria[7] and diagnosed with pSS (n = 115), sSS (n = 44), or classified as individuals with sicca symptoms (n = 50), and asymptomatic controls (n = 36). The SG-US parameters major SGs size, echogenicity, parenchymal inhomogeneity, focal changes, and posterior border were investigated using a novel US score for parenchymal inhomogeneity (0–12). Ultrasonographic abnormalities were detected in 93.0% of patients with pSS, in 27.3% with secondary SS, in 50.0% with sicca symptoms, and in 11.1% of the asymptomatic controls. Setting the SG-US inhomogeneity score cutoff at 6 resulted in the best ratio of specificity (90.0%) to sensitivity (95.1%), with a positive predictive value of 72% and a negative predictive value of 96%. The US inhomogeneity score $\geq$6 also correlated with positive biopsy and scintigraphy findings.

Finally, Luciano and colleagues[46] assessed the usefulness of SG-US in distinguishing patients with SS (n = 55) from individuals with xerostomia and/or xerophthalmia and a diagnosis of stable undifferentiated connective tissue disease (UCTD) (n = 54). Patients with SS according to the AECG criteria[7] presented a higher SG-US score compared with UCTD. Moreover, setting the SG-US cutoff greater than 2 provided a sensitivity of 65%, a specificity of 96%, a positive predictive value of 95%, and a negative predictive value of 73% for the diagnosis of SS.

On the basis of these encouraging results, the diagnostic performance of SG-US in the AECG criteria was investigated in a cohort with suspected pSS (n = 158).[14] Applying the AECG criteria[7] alone, the diagnosis of pSS presented a sensitivity of 77.9% and a specificity of 98.7% as compared with expert opinion. Compared with the AECG criteria alone, the addition of SG-US $\geq$2 to the AECG criteria, on top of autoantibodies and a positive biopsy, increased sensitivity to 87.0% but did not alter specificity (96.1% vs 98.7%). In another series of patients with suspected SS (n = 101), SG-US was found to increase also the diagnostic performance of the ACR criteria.[47] Salivary gland US was 60.0% sensitive and 87.5% specific for SS, and adding the SG-US score to the ACR criteria[8] increased sensitivity from 64.4% to 84.4% and only slightly decreased specificity from 91.1% to 89.3%.

Similar findings were presented by Takagi and colleagues,[48] who evaluated SG-US as an additional classification item in the ACR classification of SS in a cohort of 581 individuals classified as pSS (n = 364) or non-SS (n = 217) according to the AECG criteria.[7] Salivary gland US was performed in selected patients with SS (n = 102) and non-SS (n = 82), who had scored 2 or more positive or 2 or more negative results according to the ACR criteria.[8] A parotid and/or submandibular gland scored with $\geq$1 was considered positive. With the AECG criteria[7] as gold standard, ACR criteria diagnosed patients (n = 184) with 91% sensitivity, 90% specificity, and 91% accuracy. Salivary gland US alone diagnosed the ACR patients with 79% sensitivity, 90% specificity, and 83% accuracy, comparable to the results of US diagnosis in the AECG cohort (81%, 86%, and 83%, respectively). Incorporating the SG-US criteria as an alternative to 1 of the 3 ACR classification items achieved 89% to 91% sensitivity, 87% to 96% specificity, and 89% or 92% accuracy, comparable to that of the original ACR classification. Kappa analysis indicated that the original ACR and US-replaced ACR classifications matched (kappa = 0.960–0.974).

The application of a simplified scoring system has been suggested to improve interobserver and intraobserver reliability. Theander and colleagues[49] suggested to grade parenchymal homogeneity in SGs from 0 to 3, with grades 0 (normal) and 1 (mild inhomogeneity) being interpreted as normal or unspecific, and grades 2 (several rounded) and 3 (numerous or confluent hypoechoic lesions) as pSS-typical (similar to illustrated in **Fig. 3**). The authors tested the simplified score in patients with pSS (n = 105) classified according to the AECG criteria[7] and controls (n = 57), and found that the characteristic hypoechoic lesions (score 2 or 3) were observed in 52% of patients with pSS and in 1 (1.8%) of controls. Specificity and positive predictive value of abnormal SG-US for pSS were both 98%, with sensitivity and negative predictive value 52% and 53%. Theander and colleagues[49] also found that patients with pathologic SG-US had significantly more signs and symptoms of systemic complications, higher disease activity, and more frequently markers of lymphoma development, such as SG swelling, skin vasculitis, germinal center (GC)-like structures in minor SG biopsy, and CD4+ T-lymphocytopenia.

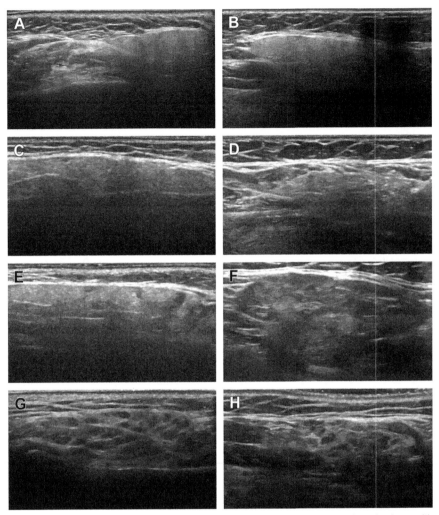

Fig. 3. Ultrasonographic images of parotid glands (*left column*; A, C, E, G) and submandibular glands (*right column*; B, D, F, H), illustrating gradual pathologic changes in parenchymal homogeneity in SGs using a simplified scoring system. The system was applied by Theander and colleagues,[49] with grades 0 (normal) (A, B) and 1 (mild inhomogeneity) (C, D) being interpreted as normal or unspecific, and grades 2 (several rounded) (E, F) and 3 (numerous or confluent hypoechoic lesions) (G, H) as typical for pSS. Hammenfors and colleagues[16] used a similar simplified scoring system previously described by Hocevar and colleagues 2005,[42] where ultrasonographic scans were graded on a scale 0 to 3, with grades 0 to 1 considered corresponding to normal/nonspecific changes (A–D) and grades 2 to 3 to pathologic changes (E–H). (*Courtesy of* Daniel Hammenfors, MD, University of Bergen, Bergen, Norway.)

Similarly Hammenfors and colleagues[16] performed SG-US in patients with pSS (n = 97), using a simplified scoring system for glandular homogeneity and hypoechogenic areas previously described by Hocevar and colleagues 2005.[42] Scans were graded on a scale 0 to 3, grades 0 to 1 considered corresponding to normal/nonspecific changes and grades 2 to 3 to pathologic changes (similar to illustrated in **Fig. 3**). Interestingly, pathologic changes were more frequent and more severe in the submandibular glands than the parotid glands. Oral and ocular sicca symptoms correlated with US score and decreased saliva levels, and patients with normal/nonspecific US findings tended to be older than patients with pathologic US findings. The US score correlated with unstimulated and stimulated salivary secretion and tear secretion. Minor SG inflammation correlated with major SG-US findings, and lymphoid organization in the form of GC-like structures in the minor SG tissue biopsies was seemingly related to pathologic changes as determined by SG-US. Serum autoantibodies against Ro/SSA and/or La/SSB were also associated with pathologic SG-US findings.

The viability of SG-US as a predictor of minor SG histology and in stratifying patients with pSS and possibly reducing the need for biopsy in patients who are negative for extractable nuclear antibody (ENA) was investigated in a cohort of patients with suspected pSS.[50] Minor SG biopsies and SG-US images were retrospectively and blindly analyzed by independent experts. In the investigated cohort, patients (n = 36) fulfilled the AECG criteria for pSS[7] or were characterized as non-SS sicca controls (n = 49). Among the patients with pSS, 16 of 36 were ENA negative, but had a positive biopsy; 14 of 16 also had a positive SG-US. The ENA-positive patients with pSS (n = 20) all had a positive SG-US, but only 15 of 20 had a positive biopsy. In 49 of 51 patients with a negative SG-US, the minor SG biopsy was also negative, indicating negative SG-US as highly predictive for a negative biopsy (96%). In 29 of 34 patients with a positive SG-US, the minor SG biopsy was positive, showing a good positive predictive value (85%) of the minor SG histology. Overall concordance between SG-US and histology was 91% (Kappa = 0.826), indicating a potential role of SG-US in stratifying ENA-negative patients, as an aid to prioritize the minor SG biopsy.

Juvenile Sjögren's Syndrome

Juvenile SS (jSS) is a rare, poorly defined and possibly underdiagnosed condition.[51,52] The disease affects children and adolescents, with mean age of diagnosis 10.7 years.[53] As in adults, a variety of organ systems may be affected in jSS, resulting in neurologic, dermatologic, musculoskeletal, vascular, gastrointestinal, respiratory, renal, and hematological manifestations.[54,55] Extraglandular manifestations have been reported with a prevalence of 51.3% in jSS.[51]

Being a rare disorder, most reports of jSS are of single cases.[56] Juvenile SS has distinctive clinical features, and diagnosis is based on clinical symptoms and presence of autoantibodies, after exclusion of infectious or lymphoproliferative diseases. Diagnosis, treatment, and follow-up of jSS is generally based on clinical experience from pSS in adults, but in comparison with pSS in adults, patients with jSS often display swelling of the major SGs as an initial symptom.[53,57] Recurrent parotitis in childhood most commonly is of infectious origin or due to retention of saliva. In jSS, parotid swelling usually precedes regular oral and ocular symptoms, whereas typical serologic findings may be absent.[56] Salivary gland US shows typical features of pSS/jSS that can add useful information, and SG-US has been suggested as a routine imaging tool in patients with recurrent parotitis and autoantibodies.[58]

Clinical presentation, diagnosis, and management of recurrent parotitis of childhood was studied to confirm a clinical pSS diagnosis.[59] Children with diseases affecting the parotid glands were retrospectively studied in a hospital cohort, and in a period of 21 years, 53 children with recurrent parotitis were identified. Interestingly, the cohort comprised more male than female patients. The age of onset was biphasic, with more patients presenting with recurrent parotitis at 2 to 5 years of age and at 10 years. Common symptoms were swelling (100%), pain (92.5%), and fever (41.5%), usually lasting 2 to 7 days with a median of 3 days. The mean frequency of symptoms was

8 episodes per year. Diagnosis was often delayed, in 70% of patients more than 1 year, to a maximum of 8 years. Common diagnoses before the definitive diagnosis of recurrent parotitis were mumps (21%), "infection" (15%), and stones (11%). Imaging modalities, such as sialogram (57%) and/or US (41%) showed sialectasis in 81% of patients. The parotitis was treated with antibiotics in more than half of the patients (54%). Final diagnoses were hypogammaglobulinemia (n = 2), human immunodeficiency virus infection (n = 1), and SS (n = 1). High-titer antinuclear antibodies (ANA) were detected in 2 children. The major clinical features distinguishing recurrent parotitis from other causes were the recurrent episodes, and the lack of pus. Clinical diagnosis often can be confirmed by SG-US and affected children should be screened for SS and immune deficiency.

In a case-report, SG-US and MRI were used to diagnose pSS in a 13-year-old girl, with a history of recurrent bilateral, parotid swelling lasting 2 years.[60] The patient history included severe arthralgia, local edema, and purpura episodes since 9 years of age. Salivary gland US and MRI of the parotid glands showed parenchymal inhomogeneity related to adipose degeneration and nodular pattern. Serologically, elevated erythrocyte sedimentation rate, the presence of hypergammaglobulinemia, positive ANA, and elevated rheumatoid factor, anti-Ro/SSA, and anti-La/SSB were detected. In the labial minor, SG biopsy focal periductal lymphocytic infiltrate and sialoduct ectasia were observed, and the patient was diagnosed with pSS.

SUMMARY AND DISCUSSION

US has become widely available for bedside, real-time imaging of the major SGs. Being user-friendly, rapidly performed, repeatable, noninvasive, and nonradiating, SG-US has emerged as a promising diagnostic and prognostic tool for pSS. The technique may also prove helpful in clinical practice to monitor patients in follow-up, and more specifically their response to therapy. With regard to treatment, Doppler has also been suggested to enable assessment of blood inflow responses to salivary stimulation. The method also appears suitable to determine the diagnosis of pSS/jSS in children with recurrent parotid swelling/parotitis.

Nonetheless, potential pitfalls remain before SG-US may come into use in clinical practice, and some of these were addressed in 2 systematic reviews.[61,62] SG-US scoring systems, the type and number of glands tested, study design, and metric properties according to OMERACT filter (truth, discrimination, and feasibility)[61] in publications from PubMed and EMBASE (January 1988–January 2013) were considered. Of the identified publications (n = 167), 31 met the inclusion criteria. Most studies had applied the AECG classification criteria for SS.[7] Ultrasonographic examination in patients with suspected pSS provided a sensitivity of 45.8% to 91.6% and a specificity of 73.0% to 98.1%. Heterogeneity was observed with regard to the definition of SG-US in B-mode, and only a few studies used color Doppler. Reliability of US and sensitivity to change in pSS was not commonly reported.

Similarly, the performance of studies was addressed in the meta-analysis by Delli and colleagues[62] who had identified 37 studies and 33 US scoring systems published until June 2014. Significant heterogeneity was detected between studies in "patient selection" (ie, pSS vs healthy volunteers, pSS vs suspected SS, or pSS vs sicca patients), "conduct and interpretation of ultrasonography," and "flow of patients and timing of tests." The investigators concluded that the quality of available studies was low, not allowing the assessment of SG-US as a reliable and practical tool in diagnosing SS.

Taken together, further studies are warranted to validate and standardize the US definition of SG in pSS. First, consensus for a standardized procedure and validated common scoring system must be established, to increase the intraobserver and inter-observer reproducibility and to better assess the value of SG-US in patient monitoring and follow-up. Once validated, the novel common scoring system should be tested in larger disease-controlled studies, to redefine the specificity of SG-US in the diagnostic algorithm of SS. Whereas the scientific community is opening new venues for the use of SG-US in the diagnosis of SS, other possible applications for SG-US are on the horizon, such as an aid to recognize different subsets of pSS patients and especially those at risk for lymphoma development.

REFERENCES

1. Jonsson R, Kroneld U, Backman K, et al. Progression of sialadenitis in Sjögren's syndrome. Br J Rheumatol 1993;32(7):578–81.
2. Jonsson R, Bowman SJ, Gordon TP. Sjögren's syndrome. In: Koopman WJ, editor. Arthritis and allied conditions. 15th edition. Philadelphia: Lippincott Williams & Wilkins; 2005. p. 1681–705.
3. Mengshoel AM, Norheim KB, Omdal R. Primary Sjögren's syndrome: fatigue is an ever-present, fluctuating, and uncontrollable lack of energy. Arthritis Care Res 2014;66(8):1227–32.
4. Johnsen SJ, Brun JG, Goransson LG, et al. Risk of non-Hodgkin's lymphoma in primary Sjögren's syndrome: a population-based study. Arthritis Care Res 2013;65(5):816–21.
5. Voulgarelis M, Dafni UG, Isenberg DA, et al. Malignant lymphoma in primary Sjögren's syndrome: a multicenter, retrospective, clinical study by the European Concerted Action on Sjögren's Syndrome. Arthritis Rheum 1999; 42(8):1765–72.
6. Theander E, Henriksson G, Ljungberg O, et al. Lymphoma and other malignancies in primary Sjögren's syndrome: a cohort study on cancer incidence and lymphoma predictors. Ann Rheum Dis 2006;65(6):796–803.
7. Vitali C, Bombardieri S, Jonsson R, et al. Classification criteria for Sjögren's syndrome: a revised version of the European criteria proposed by the American-European Consensus Group. Ann Rheum Dis 2002;61(6):554–8.
8. Shiboski SC, Shiboski CH, Criswell LA, et al. American College of Rheumatology classification criteria for Sjögren's syndrome: a data-driven, expert consensus approach in the Sjögren's International Collaborative Clinical Alliance Cohort. Arthritis Care Res 2012;64(4):475–87.
9. Shiboski CH, Shiboski SC, Group A-ESsSCCW. Proposed ACR-EULAR classification criteria for Sjögren's syndrome: development and validation. 15th International Symposium on Sjögren's Syndrome; Bergen (Norway). Scand J Immunol 2015;330.
10. Shiboski CH. Development and validation of ACR-EULAR classification criteria for Sjögren's syndrome. New ACR-EULAR Sjögren's Syndrome Classification Criteria and Updates. [Invited communication], in press.
11. Obinata K, Sato T, Ohmori K, et al. A comparison of diagnostic tools for Sjögren syndrome, with emphasis on sialography, histopathology, and ultrasonography. Oral Surg Oral Med Oral Pathol Oral Radiol Endod 2010;109(1):129–34.
12. De Vita S, Lorenzon G, Rossi G, et al. Salivary gland echography in primary and secondary Sjögren's syndrome. Clin Exp Rheumatol 1992;10(4):351–6.
13. Wernicke D, Hess H, Gromnica-Ihle E, et al. Ultrasonography of salivary glands–a highly specific imaging procedure for diagnosis of Sjögren's syndrome. J Rheumatol 2008;35(2):285–93.

14. Cornec D, Jousse-Joulin S, Pers JO, et al. Contribution of salivary gland ultrasonography to the diagnosis of Sjögren's syndrome: toward new diagnostic criteria? Arthritis Rheum 2013;65(1):216–25.
15. Lindvall AM, Jonsson R. The salivary gland component of Sjögren's syndrome: an evaluation of diagnostic methods. Oral Surg Oral Med Oral Pathol 1986;62(1):32–42.
16. Hammenfors DS, Brun JG, Jonsson R, et al. Diagnostic utility of major salivary gland ultrasonography in primary Sjögren's syndrome. Clin Exp Rheumatol 2015;33(1):56–62.
17. Rubin P, Holt JF. Secretory sialography in diseases of the major salivary glands. Am J Roentgenol Radium Ther Nucl Med 1957;77(4):575–98.
18. Whaley K, Blair S, Low PS, et al. Sialographic abnormalities in Sjögren's syndrome, rheumatoid arthritis, and other arthritides and connective tissue diseases. A clinical and radiological investigation using hydrostatic sialography. Clin Radiol 1972;23(4):474–82.
19. Astreinidou E, Roesink JM, Raaijmakers CP, et al. 3D MR sialography as a tool to investigate radiation-induced xerostomia: feasibility study. Int J Radiat Oncol Biol Phys 2007;68(5):1310–9.
20. Shimizu M, Okamura K, Yoshiura K, et al. Sonographic diagnostic criteria for screening Sjögren's syndrome. Oral Surg Oral Med Oral Pathol Oral Radiol Endod 2006;102(1):85–93.
21. Fujibayashi T, Sugai S, Miyasaka N, et al. Revised Japanese criteria for Sjögren's syndrome (1999): availability and validity. Mod Rheumatol 2004;14(6):425–34.
22. Chikui T, Okamura K, Tokumori K, et al. Quantitative analyses of sonographic images of the parotid gland in patients with Sjögren's syndrome. Ultrasound Med Biol 2006;32(5):617–22.
23. Chikui T, Shimizu M, Kawazu T, et al. A quantitative analysis of sonographic images of the salivary gland: a comparison between sonographic and sialographic findings. Ultrasound Med Biol 2009;35(8):1257–64.
24. Poul JH, Brown JE, Davies J. Retrospective study of the effectiveness of high-resolution ultrasound compared with sialography in the diagnosis of Sjögren's syndrome. Dentomaxillofac Radiol 2008;37(7):392–7.
25. Takagi Y, Kimura Y, Nakamura H, et al. Salivary gland ultrasonography: can it be an alternative to sialography as an imaging modality for Sjögren's syndrome? Ann Rheum Dis 2010;69(7):1321–4.
26. Song GG, Lee YH. Diagnostic accuracies of sialography and salivary ultrasonography in Sjögren's syndrome patients: a meta-analysis. Clin Exp Rheumatol 2014;32(4):516–22.
27. Decuzzi M, Tatulli F, Giampaolo M, et al. Sialocintigraphy versus ultrasonography of the salivary glands in patients first diagnosed with Sjögren's syndrome. Hell J Nucl Med 2006;9(2):103–5.
28. Salaffi F, Carotti M, Iagnocco A, et al. Ultrasonography of salivary glands in primary Sjögren's syndrome: a comparison with contrast sialography and scintigraphy. Rheumatology (Oxford) 2008;47(8):1244–9.
29. Milic VD, Petrovic RR, Boricic IV, et al. Diagnostic value of salivary gland ultrasonographic scoring system in primary Sjögren's syndrome: a comparison with scintigraphy and biopsy. J Rheumatol 2009;36(7):1495–500.
30. Milic V, Petrovic R, Boricic I, et al. Ultrasonography of major salivary glands could be an alternative tool to sialoscintigraphy in the American-European classification criteria for primary Sjögren's syndrome. Rheumatology (Oxford) 2012;51(6):1081–5.

31. Wu CB, Xi H, Zhou Q, et al. The diagnostic value of technetium 99m pertechnetate salivary gland scintigraphy in patients with certain salivary gland diseases. J Oral Maxillofac Surg 2015;73(3):443–50.

32. Carotti M, Ciapetti A, Jousse-Joulin S, et al. Ultrasonography of the salivary glands: the role of grey-scale and colour/power Doppler. Clin Exp Rheumatol 2014;32(1 Suppl 80):S61–70.

33. Jousse-Joulin S, Devauchelle-Pensec V, Morvan J, et al. Ultrasound assessment of salivary glands in patients with primary Sjögren's syndrome treated with rituximab: quantitative and Doppler waveform analysis. Biologics 2007;1(3):311–9.

34. Jousse-Joulin S, Devauchelle-Pensec V, Cornec D, et al. Brief report: ultrasonographic assessment of salivary gland response to rituximab in primary Sjögren's syndrome. Arthritis Rheum 2015;67(6):1623–8.

35. Shimizu M, Okamura K, Yoshiura K, et al. Sonographic diagnosis of Sjögren syndrome: evaluation of parotid gland vascularity as a diagnostic tool. Oral Surg Oral Med Oral Pathol Oral Radiol Endod 2008;106(4):587–94.

36. Giuseppetti GM, Argalia G, Salera D, et al. Ultrasonographic contrast-enhanced study of sicca syndrome. Eur J Radiol 2005;54(2):225–32.

37. Ophir J, Cespedes I, Ponnekanti H, et al. Elastography: a quantitative method for imaging the elasticity of biological tissues. Ultrason Imaging 1991;13(2):111–34.

38. Dejaco C, De Zordo T, Heber D, et al. Real-time sonoelastography of salivary glands for diagnosis and functional assessment of primary Sjögren's syndrome. Ultrasound Med Biol 2014;40(12):2759–67.

39. Samier-Guerin A, Saraux A, Gestin S, et al. Can ARFI elastometry of the salivary glands contribute to the diagnosis of Sjögren's syndrome? Joint Bone Spine 2015. [Epub ahead of print].

40. Zhang S, Zhu J, Zhang X, et al. Assessment of the Stiffness of Major Salivary Glands in Primary Sjögren's Syndrome through Quantitative Acoustic Radiation Force Impulse Imaging. Ultrasound Med Biol 2016;42(3):645–53.

41. Manthorpe R, Oxholm P, Prause JU, et al. The Copenhagen criteria for Sjögren's syndrome. Scand J Rheumatol Suppl 1986;61:19–21.

42. Hocevar A, Ambrozic A, Rozman B, et al. Ultrasonographic changes of major salivary glands in primary Sjögren's syndrome. Diagnostic value of a novel oooring oyotom. Rheumatology (Oxford) 2005;44(6):768–72.

43. Hocevar A, Rainer S, Rozman B, et al. Ultrasonographic changes of major salivary glands in primary Sjögren's syndrome. Evaluation of a novel scoring system. Eur J Radiol 2007;63(3):379–83.

44. Baldini C, Luciano N, Tarantini G, et al. Salivary gland ultrasonography: a highly specific tool for the early diagnosis of primary Sjögren's syndrome. Arthritis Res Ther 2015;17:146.

45. Milic VD, Petrovic RR, Boricic IV, et al. Major salivary gland sonography in Sjögren's syndrome: diagnostic value of a novel ultrasonography score (0-12) for parenchymal inhomogeneity. Scand J Rheumatol 2010;39(2):160–6.

46. Luciano N, Baldini C, Tarantini G, et al. Ultrasonography of major salivary glands: a highly specific tool for distinguishing primary Sjögren's syndrome from undifferentiated connective tissue diseases. Rheumatology (Oxford) 2015;54(12):2198–204.

47. Cornec D, Jousse-Joulin S, Marhadour T, et al. Salivary gland ultrasonography improves the diagnostic performance of the 2012 American College of Rheumatology classification criteria for Sjögren's syndrome. Rheumatology (Oxford) 2014;53(9):1604–7.

48. Takagi Y, Sumi M, Nakamura H, et al. Salivary gland ultrasonography as a primary imaging tool for predicting efficacy of xerostomia treatment in patients with Sjögren's syndrome. Rheumatology (Oxford) 2015;55(2):237–45.

49. Theander E, Mandl T. Primary Sjögren's syndrome: the diagnostic and prognostic value of salivary gland ultrasonography using a simplified scoring system. Arthritis Care Res 2014;66(7):1102–7.

50. Astorri E, Sutcliffe N, Richards PS, et al. Ultrasound of the salivary glands is a strong predictor of labial gland biopsy histopathology in patients with sicca symptoms. J Oral Pathol Med 2015. [Epub ahead of print].

51. Anaya JM, Ogawa N, Talal N. Sjögren's syndrome in childhood. J Rheumatol 1995;22(6):1152–8.

52. Lieberman SM. Childhood Sjögren syndrome: insights from adults and animal models. Curr Opin Rheumatol 2013;25(5):651–7.

53. Cimaz R, Casadei A, Rose C, et al. Primary Sjögren syndrome in the paediatric age: a multicentre survey. Eur J Pediatr 2003;162(10):661–5.

54. Nikitakis NG, Rivera H, Lariccia C, et al. Primary Sjögren syndrome in childhood: report of a case and review of the literature. Oral Surg Oral Med Oral Pathol Oral Radiol Endod 2003;96(1):42–7.

55. Bogdanovic R, Basta-Jovanovic G, Putnik J, et al. Renal involvement in primary Sjögren syndrome of childhood: case report and literature review. Mod Rheumatol 2013;23(1):182–9.

56. de Souza TR, Silva IH, Carvalho AT, et al. Juvenile Sjögren syndrome: distinctive age, unique findings. Pediatr Dent 2012;34(5):427–30.

57. Fang QG, Liu FY, Sun CF. Recurrent submandibular gland swelling as a first manifestation in a child with primary Sjögren syndrome. J Craniofac Surg 2013;24(4): e413–5.

58. Nieto-Gonzalez JC, Monteagudo I, Bello N, et al. Salivary gland ultrasound in children: a useful tool in the diagnosis of juvenile Sjögren's syndrome. Clin Exp Rheumatol 2014;32(4):578–80.

59. Leerdam CM, Martin HC, Isaacs D. Recurrent parotitis of childhood. J Paediatr Child Health 2005;41(12):631–4.

60. Civilibal M, Canpolat N, Yurt A, et al. A child with primary Sjögren syndrome and a review of the literature. Clin Pediatr (Phila) 2007;46(8):738–42.

61. Jousse-Joulin S, Milic V, Jonsson MV, et al. Is salivary gland ultrasonography a useful tool in Sjögren's syndrome? A systematic review. Rheumatology (Oxford) 2016;55(5):789–800.

62. Delli K, Dijkstra PU, Stel AJ, et al. Diagnostic properties of ultrasound of major salivary glands in Sjögren's syndrome: a meta-analysis. Oral Dis 2015;21(6): 792–800.

Sjögren Syndrome
Why Do Clinical Trials Fail?

Robert I. Fox, MD, PhD*, Carla M. Fox, RN

KEYWORDS

- Sjögren syndrome • Benign glandular manifestations
- Extraglandular manifestations • Keratoconjunctivitis sicca • Danger hypothesis
- Danger-associated molecular patterns • Functional circuit
- Neurohypothalamic-immune axis

KEY POINTS

- Failure of benign manifestations, such as fatigue or cognitive impairment, must be shown by current peripheral blood tests.
- Benign symptoms, including dry eye and dry mouth, correlate poorly with objective findings of tear flow and saliva flow.
- Many of Sjögren syndrome patients who have extraglandular manifestations are incorrectly labeled as systemic lupus erythematosus or rheumatoid arthritis patients.

INTRODUCTION

Symptoms of Sjögren syndrome (SS) include both benign and systemic manifestations.

The benign (glandular) symptoms include ocular and oral discomfort. The myalgias and arthralgias, as well as generalized fatigue and cognitive difficulties, are also included in the benign category. However, these features certainly are not benign to the patients.[1–3]

Dry or painful eyes are now the most frequent reason for visits to ophthalmology clinic, and a leading cause of lost work efficiency.

Because patients increasingly sit at computer stations in low-humidity office buildings, tear film dysfunction is exacerbated by the 90% blink rate reduction that accompanies staring at the computer screen.[4]

In the United Kingdom alone, the financial loss from dry eyes alone was estimated at more than £150,000,000.[3,5]

Patients' most commonly identified benign symptom limiting their daily function is the chronic fatigue and loss of ability to function at their previous cognitive level.

Rheumatology Clinic, Scripps Memorial Hospital, XiMED Medical Group, 9850 Genesee Avenue, Suite 910, La Jolla, CA 92037, USA
* Corresponding author.
E-mail address: robertfoxmd@mac.com

Rheum Dis Clin N Am 42 (2016) 519–530
http://dx.doi.org/10.1016/j.rdc.2016.03.009
0889-857X/16/$ – see front matter © 2016 Elsevier Inc. All rights reserved.

rheumatic.theclinics.com

The patients equate this disability at the level of moderate angina, and state that they would be willing to exchange more than 2 years of life expectancy to not have this limitation.[6]

The benign symptoms emphasized here are benign only in their nomenclature; these have been the symptoms that have not shown improvements in clinical trials with biologic agents.[7,8]

Yet, rheumatologists and investigators have assumed that the next anticytokine therapy will have a different and better result than the numerous other anticytokine therapies that are buried in the graveyard of failed clinical trials over the past decade.

The future of therapy for SS is not that bleak but clinicians and investigators must stop and ask about the choice of targets, methods of biomarkers, and trial design.

- If extraglandular manifestations of SS are going to be targeted, suitable SS patients must be identified and more efficiently enrolled. This involves education of rheumatologists and other specialists about sick SS patients misclassified as systemic lupus erythematosus (SLE) or rheumatoid arthritis (RA) patients.
- If benign symptoms are going to be targeted, neurochemists have much to teach about the pathways that mediate these symptoms. A broader understanding of the innate immune system and how it interacts with the central immune system is provided by murine sickness models after viral infection.

BACKGROUND

To consider the future of therapy in SS, the concept of the danger hypothesis that gave rise to exploration of the innate immune system and its interactions with the central nervous system (CNS) is reviewed (**Box 1**).[9–14]

This hypothesis includes the traditional adaptive or acquired immune system of T-cell–mediated B-cell production of autoantibodies. However, it also includes the interactions of the innate immune system with elements of the CNS.

The adaptive (or acquired) immune system is based on Medewar's failure of tolerance model, and has provided a family of drugs used to treat the extraglandular manifestations of SS, including disease-modifying antirheumatic drugs (DMARDs) and many biologic drugs.

However, it was recognized more than 25 years ago that the adaptive peripheral immune system did not adequately explain the interaction of the peripheral immune system with the CNS. A broader immune system was proposed to distinguish self from exogenous infections, as outlined by the danger model hypothesis of Gallucci and Matzinger[10] and Janeway and Medzhitov[12,14] (see **Box 1**).

In the danger model, the peripheral innate immune system still provides the first line of defense but subsequently interacts with the midbrain, the cerebral cortex, and the hypothalamic-adrenal axis by a series of danger-associated molecular patterns (DAMPs) leading to up regulation of toll-like receptors (TLRs) in activated astroglial cells. This activation results in up regulation of neurohormones, cytokines, neurokines, prostaglandins, and neurotransmitters. Morris and colleagues[15] have recently summarized the interactions between activation of DAMPs and central mechanisms of fatigue that involve pathways of tumor necrosis factor (TNF), interferon (IFN)-1 and -2, and ultimately mitochondrial processing of ATP. This is shown schematically in **Fig. 1**.[15]

REASONS FOR FAILURE OF TRIALS OF BIOLOGICS IN SJÖGREN SYNDROME TRIALS

It is important to point out that there has not been total failure of biologics in SS. Reasonable results in the control of extraglandular manifestations of SS have been achieved.

Box 1
Models of autoimmune disease: tolerance model and danger signal

The initial development of development of disease-modifying antirheumatic drugs (DMARDs) and immunosuppressive drugs was based on the identification of autoantibodies in subjects and rejection of skin grafts in animals or humans. This led to recognition of human leukocyte antigens, T-cells, and B-cells. This led to the tolerance model.

To explain the ability of the immune system to distinguish self from modified self, the role of the thymus in removing self-reactive lymphocytes was recognized by Medawar.[9] For those self-reactive lymphocytes that escaped thymic deletion, autoimmune disease was the consequence. The thymus was an organ in which almost all new lymphocytes underwent apoptosis and any lymphocytes reactive with these self-products were destined for self-death.

In Medawar's tolerance model, a back-up system of peripheral immune suppression of lymphocytes was proposed to eliminate autoimmune cells that managed to sneak through thymic screening. Autoimmune disease was a failure of these mechanisms and therapy was directed to correcting these immune lapses. Therapy directed by this model led to great success in organ graft transplantation and certain autoimmune disorders.

Subsequently, it would be recognized that the tolerance mechanisms of the immune system (ie, acquired or adaptive immune system) evolved later than a more primitive innate immune system. However, this model guided immunologic studies and therapy for more than 2 decades.

Initial therapies, including steroids, DMARDs, and immune suppressive drugs, were developed using these models. However, the products of activation of the acquired immune system (eg, cytokine or autoantibody levels) remain the main sources of outcome markers in therapeutic trials.

Although elegant, the tolerance model did not explain many of the observed immediate responses of the immune system or the overall changes in behavior that accompanied immune challenge. A more general danger signal hypothesis was proposed by Gallucci and Matzinger,[10] Janeway and Medzhitov,[12,14] and Medzhitov and Janeway.[11,13] The danger system model incorporated the adrenal hypothalamic axis and the role of prostaglandins, as well as the role of cortical (CNS) memory in the form of danger signals, in addition to immune responses of adaptive memory lymphocytes.

The key extension of the danger system model was the multiorgan responses needed to recognize and respond to infections. This predicted and incorporated the innate immune system in the periphery, including TLR receptors. It further predicted the CNS communication with the peripheral immune system. However, markers that correlate with the complex CNS changes that accompany response to foreign infections or autoimmune diseases that mimic these reactions have yet to be identified.

An understanding of the danger model and its markers will represent the therapeutic challenge of the next decade

Tolerance model (distinguish self from altered-self at thymic level)[a]

- Human leukocyte antigens
- T-cells and specific antigen driven responses
- Costimulatory factors
- B-cells and autoantibodies
- Memory at level of peripheral immune system

Danger signal model (distinguish self from infection)[b]

- Peripheral immune system communicates with CNS
- Innate toll-like receptors in periphery
- Unique toll-like receptors in CNS
- Cytokines, neurokines, neurotransmitters

- Prostaglandins and lipoproteins
- Hypothalamic, adrenal axis
- CNS and peripheral nervous system modulation of inflammation
- Memory at cortical level of danger signals

[a]Medawar[9]
[b]Gallucci and Matzinger,[10] Matzinger and Janeway,[11,13] and Janeway and Matzinger[12,14]

Indeed, the most widely used biologic agent for treatment of SS in Europe is rituximab,[16–19] although it is not yet approved for SS in the United States by the Food and Drug Administration (FDA).

The failure for FDA approval of rituximab derives from the failure of biologic agents to improve SS benign symptoms and the relatively small proportion of SS patients with extraglandular symptoms in the pivotal double-blind trials.[20]

A PubMed literature search reveals more than 5000 published studies (including many double-blind studies) on the use of rituximab and other biologic agents in extraglandular manifestations of SS.

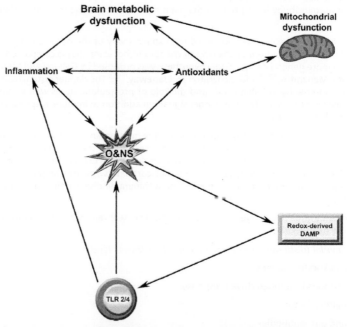

Fig. 1. Prolonged and or excessive stimulation of membrane-bound TLRs results in the production of proinflammatory cytokines and reactive oxygen and nitrogen species (ROS/RNS) to cause macromolecule damage leading to the production of redox-derived DAMPs. The presence of such DAMPs leads to chronic engagement of TLRs and a spiraling, self-amplifying pattern of increasing ROS/RNS. Increasing levels of ROS/RNS damage mitochondrial lipids and proteins, leading to dissipation of the mitochondrial membrane, inhibition of the electron transport chain, activation of microglia, and astrocytes in the brain. NS, nitrous oxide species; O, oxygen radical. (*From* Morris G, Berk M, Walder K, et al. Central pathways causing fatigue in neuroinflammatory and autoimmune illnesses. BMC Med 2015;13:28.)

However, rituximab was not given on a routine preventive schedule in these published studies but was given in response to particular manifestations such as vasculitis, mixed cryoglobulinemia, intractable rashes, or other organ involvement.

This is not a heretical suggestion because infections are not treated on a prophylactic basis but after the signs and symptoms are present.

Unfortunately, SS subjects with a high level of EULAR Sjögren Syndrome Disease Activity Index (ESSDAI) are not numerous enough or are often clinically unsuitable for the type of prospective randomized study required for approval in the United States by the FDA.

Among studies of other biologic agents, such as abatacept (Orencia) or belimumab (Benlysta), that have been presented in publication or abstract form, improvements of ESSDAI of 3.5 or more have been achieved.[21–24]

However, the length of time to enroll and randomize an adequate number of these subjects with such active disease has been quite long, suggesting that the use of this drug in most SS patients would be impractical.

Further, the level of improvement in the patient's quality of life assessment in most belimumab-treated patients was not improved sufficiently to consider these medications cost-effective or gain approval to formulary in Europe. In the United States, where the drug is approved for SLE, the enthusiasm for the drug by both patients and rheumatologists has been limited.

MAJOR PROBLEM IN ENROLLING SJÖGREN SYNDROME PATIENTS WITH EXTRAGLANDULAR MANIFESTATIONS: MANY OF THE SICKEST SJÖGREN SYNDROME PATIENTS ARE MISCLASSIFIED AS SYSTEMIC LUPUS ERYTHEMATOSUS, RHEUMATOID ARTHRITIS, OR PROGRESSIVE SYSTEMIC SCLEROSIS

An important recent presentation at the 2015 American College of Rheumatology (ACR) conference by Rasmussen and colleagues[25] pointed out that more than half of the sickest SS patients were incorrectly diagnosed as SLE or RA (http://acrabstracts.org/abstract/previous-diagnosis-of-sjogrens-syndrome-as-rheumatoid-arthritis-or-systemic-lupus-erythematosus).

Thus, even in rheumatology clinics with great expertise in diagnosing SS, the SS patients with extraglandular manifestations such as arthritis, lymphadenopathy, Idiopathic thrombocytopenic purpura (ITP), or mixed cryoglobulinemia who would be expected to benefit from biologic agents were not included in the cohort recruited for the clinical studies.

Thus, in general practice, it is not hard to imagine that the sickest SS patients are being seen in other clinics such as hematology (ITP, hemolytic anemia, lymphadenopathy), pulmonary (interstitial pneumonitis), neurology (transverse myelitis, peripheral neuropathy, mononeuritis multiplex), or renal (interstitial nephritis). These SS patients would not be correctly identified as eligible for treatment in the biologic drug trials.

Recent informal surveys among neurologists and hematologists at the authors' institution found the following:

- It is rare that a previously diagnosed SLE or RA patient who is referred to one of these other clinics for treatment of significant extraglandular manifestation with a positive antinuclear antibody (ANA) is asked about the simplest manifestations of SS to make the correct diagnosis.
- To extend these somewhat surprising results, the authors were allowed to conduct a simple informal survey of hematologists attending the American Society of Hematology meetings held in San Diego last year.
- Over 80% of these board-certified hematologists were not aware that SS antigen-A (SS-A) or SS antigen-B were not criteria for diagnosis of SLE.

The authors doubt that other specialists, including many in rheumatology, would do much better.

A PRACTICAL METHOD TO IMPROVE DIAGNOSIS OF SJÖGREN SYNDROME PATIENTS

Perhaps the easiest way to capture this sickest SS population is to concentrate on the clinical report of the ANA and rheumatoid factor (RF), which are the usual ways that patients get classified as either SLE or RA.

The gold standard for the ANA is immunofluorescent assay using a human epithelial type 2 (HEp-2) cell[26]:

- The footnote to the usual positive ANA says suggestive of SLE; however, this should be changed to SLE or SS.
- The footnote to a positive RF says RA when it should also include SS, SLE, and other causes, including infectious diseases.

It is also important to consider the causes of a false-negative ANA. Two important variables need to be considered:

1. The SS-A antigen is quite labile during fixation and, thus, a false-negative ANA will result.[27,28]
   a. Indeed, the entire clinical diagnosis of subacute lupus disappeared when it was recognized as a laboratory artifact that, over acetone fixation of substrate, caused a false-negative ANA.[29]
   b. The detection of specific antibodies such as SS-A is generally ordered by physicians as a reflex to a positive ANA and, thus, will not be ordered if the screening ANA is negative.[30–33]
      i. To overcome this problem, a specific substrate called HEp2000 was developed by transfecting a traditional HEp-2 cell with 60 kD SS-A to insure sufficient levels of antigen for detection.[34]
      ii. However, many of the large commercial laboratories do not use the HEp2000. The reason for this practice may include the apparent increased cost of using this licensed cell line in an era of cutting costs for clinical laboratory tests and, thus, SS patients are missed in screening.[35]
2. An extension of this streamlining of ANA tests has been the introduction of the enzyme-linked immunosorbent assay (ELIOA) that may not detect antigens that are relatively infrequent or denatured while preparing the ELISA substrate.[32,33]
   a. An interesting example of the discrepancy of ANA by Immunofluorescent assay (IFA) and ELISA tests is a recent clinical-pathologic conference reported on in the New England Journal of Medicine, in which the diagnosis of SLE was originally discarded, based on a negative ANA by ELISA.[36]
   b. The definitive procedure (always suggested by the alert medical student on the case) was to repeat the ANA by IFA. The correct diagnosis was then made, followed by the discussion of artefacts associated with ELISA assays.[36]

THE MECHANISMS OF FATIGUE

Perhaps fatigue and cognitive changes are the most challenging frontier for research because they accompany a variety of conditions, ranging from depression to demyelinating disorders.

Given the failure to understand why normal individuals feel these symptoms accompanying a viral flu-like illness, the most likely explanation is that the correct biomarkers are not being measured in the sampling of CNS in the peripheral blood.

In this world of medicine, if the marker cannot be measured, then the condition must not exist.

In murine models of severe fatigue after viral infection,[37] traditional peripheral biomarkers of the acquired immune system, such as erythrocyte sedimentation rate (ESR) or C-reactive protein (CRP), are not altered. These animals show change of mood, loss of grooming, increased thirst, impairment of problem solving, and social withdrawal.

The behavior of fatigue was associated in the brain by specific neural signals that activate oxidative or nitrosative (reactive nitrogen species [ROS]) stress pathways.[38–40]

The cytokine events initially identified were related to interleukin (IL)-1 and prostaglandin pathways, similar to those noted in juvenile inflammatory arthritis (JIA) and multiple sclerosis. Indeed, this pathway was the basis for therapy with fingolimod[41] in multiple sclerosis and several anti-IL-1 therapies currently used in JIA.

Although not generally discussed by rheumatologists as a part of the innate immune system, other disciplines of neurochemistry recognize this new arm of the central immune innate immune system involving TLR2/4 signaling pathway to fatigue, and use it as a model for drug development.[42]

Although the danger hypothesis was defined by the pivotal studies of Gallucci and Matzinger[10] and Janeway and Medzhitov[12,14] in mouse models of inflammation more than 20 years ago, it has escaped the central attention of rheumatology research.

At a cellular level, activation of the danger pathway responds to potential pathogens through a defined series of TLRs. The signals from the peripheral to the CNS through either cytokines, such as IL-1 or IL-6, or prostaglandin pathways.

As shown in **Fig. 1**, either pathway leads to activation of quiescent microglial cells. The activated microglial cells express a series of molecules (ie, DAMPs) and oxidative reactive species. In either case, these molecules may provide a biomarker for monitoring symptoms and new targets for therapy.

Further details of the cascade of DAMPs and oxidative reactive species that influence mitochondrial function and brain function are shown in Appendix 1.[15]

Another of the most interesting presentations at the 2015 ACR meeting, by Bårdsen and colleagues,[43] was the report that plasma levels of several cerebral spinal fluid proteins, including N-methyl-d-aspartate receptors and heat shock protein (HSP) 90, were significantly higher in patients with high fatigue compared with those SS patients with low fatigue (http://www.acrabstracts.org/abstract/serum-and-csf-biomarkers-of-neuropsychiatric-involvement-in-primary-sjogren-syndrome-and-systemic-lupus-erythematosus).

The more detailed findings on elevation of HSP90 but not HSP32 and HSP60 are currently in press.[43,44]

Thus, new markers for objectively measuring inflammatory fatigue must be validated and then incorporated in patient inclusion criteria and outcome measures to help separate this SS manifestation from a secondary depression.

THE FUNCTIONAL CIRCUIT

To understand past failures of therapy and design new therapies, a concept called the functional circuit that explains the discordance between objective findings and subjective complaints must be reviewed.[45,46]

This is shown in Appendix 1, in which unmyelinated afferent nerves leave the ocular surface in route to the midbrain (lacrimatory nuclei).

The amplification of neural signals in the midbrain under the influence of immune stimulation is the key step that has been shown in animal model (thrombospondin knockout mouse)[47] of SS to play a key step in pathogenesis.

The signals from the midbrain are reflected to areas of the cortex that can be identified by functional MRI.[48]

The efferent signals from the different regions of the cortex, including memory regions, are then sent back to the lacrimatory nuclei.

It is at that juncture that a net decision to respond is activated by sending sympathetic signals to the blood vessels, and activating G-coupled proteins and cholinergic or vasoactive intestinal peptide signals to the glandular tissue to stimulate aquaporin-mediated calcium and water movement across the acinar cell membrane.

SUMMARY

A common misconception is dryness in SS results from the total destruction of the salivary or lacrimal gland. Indeed, many SS patients with long-stranding severe sicca disease have minor or major gland biopsies that show almost 50% of the acinar and ductal tissue intact.[49,50] Additionally, the residual gland is dysfunctional with neural innervation still largely intact[51] but an electron microscopic and immunohistologic appearance demonstrate dysfunction and nonfunctional innervation.

Thus, the phone is ringing at the level of the gland but no one is answering.

To understand the failures in therapeutic trials of DMARDs and biologic agents, it is necessary to step back and consider the following:

- Although the extraglandular manifestations of the disease (ie, ESSDAI) have been improved with biologic agents, the proportion of SS patients in these studies with a very high ESSDAI is small.
- Additional SS patients with extraglandular manifestations may benefit from therapy, but they are not included in the trials because they are mislabeled as either SLE or RA.
- Clinical trials have not significantly improved benign manifestations (sicca and fatigue) that are present in most SS patients.
- Serologic markers have not been developed to reflect the impact of peripheral immune activity on the CNS
- If the conception of immune activity as outlined by the danger hypothesis is broadened, markers that reflect alterations in DAMPs (HSPs), prostaglandins, and other markers of CNS response to peripheral inflammation can be identified.
- The failure to understand and quantitate the mechanisms of benign symptoms has also led to failure of trials of biological agents in SLE, as recently reviewed by Isenberg and Merrill.[44]

Summary points
1. Some rheumatologists do not accept disabling benign symptoms described by the patient as real because they are not correlated with acute-phase reactant elevations (ie, ESR, CRP). These symptoms are dismissed as depression or fibromyalgia without considering the potential role of immune factors that influence CNS behavior in these processes.
2. Although there is dismissal of chronic fatigue in SS patients, there is a significant lack of understanding about the mechanisms that mediate fatigue and myalgia in normal individuals during a viral illness, even though their acute phase reactants are normal.
3. There is an immune causality of fatigue in patients with multiple sclerosis or Parkinson disease, even though there are not good peripheral blood markers.

4. Rheumatology literature does not report advances in recent studies in mouse models of viral illness. These animals develop sickness behavior in the absence of acute phase reactants.
5. These murine models may provide peripheral blood markers (ie, DAMPs) such as HSPs and products of prostaglandin or oxidative damage-mediated pathways.
6. In particular, murine models of sickness behavior demonstrate how peripheral immune activation leads to stimulation of microglial cells that subsequently upregulate DAMPs, and influence serotonergic and other neurokines to modulate the hypothalamic-adrenal axis and prostaglandin mechanisms.
7. The danger hypothesis, first proposed more than 25 years ago, is reviewed because it brings together these concepts.

Benign symptoms: dry eye and dry mouth correlate poorly with objective finding of tear flow and saliva flow

1. Symptoms from afferent neurons from eye and mouth may be amplified at level of midbrain (lacrimatory or salivatory nuclei). These afferent signals are then sent to different regions of the cerebral cortex.
2. Cortical processing of these ocular and oral signals is an important Darwinian trait, given the importance in survival of vision and eating.
3. The concept of the functional circuit incorporates the inflammation at the mucosal surfaces, the neural pathways that ultimately lead to the brain cortex, and the efferent neural pathways that stimulate secretory glands.

Treatment of extraglandular manifestations

1. Patients with high ESSDAI scores (a cumulative aggregate of extraglandular activity) have shown significant response to biologic agents.
   a. However, SS patients with high levels of ESSDAI are difficult to recruit into a prospective double-blind study.
2. Many of the SS patients who have extraglandular manifestations are incorrectly labeled as either SLE or RA patients.
3. Thus, the sickest SS patients and those SS patients most likely to show response to biologic agents are mislabeled and not enrolled in the studies in which they might show benefit.

REFERENCES

1. Seror R, Theander E, Bootsma H, et al. Outcome measures for primary Sjögren's syndrome: a comprehensive review. J Autoimmun 2014;51:51–6.
2. Ng W-F, Bowman SJ. Primary Sjögren's syndrome: too dry and too tired. Rheumatology 2010;49:844–53.
3. Bowman SJ, Pierre YS, Sutcliffe N, et al. Estimating indirect costs in primary Sjögren's syndrome. J Rheumatol 2010;37:1010–5.
4. Tsubota K, Nakamori K. Dry eyes and video display terminals. N Engl J Med 1993;328:584.
5. Reddy P, Grad O, Rajagopalan K. The economic burden of dry eye: a conceptual framework and preliminary assessment. Cornea 2004;23:751–61.
6. Reynolds KJ, Vernon SD, Bouchery E, et al. The economic impact of chronic fatigue syndrome. Cost Eff Resour Alloc 2004;2:4.
7. Bowman S. Biologic therapies in primary Sjögren's syndrome. Curr Pharm Biotechnol 2012;13:1997–2008.

8. Dass S, Bowman SJ, Vital EM, et al. Reduction of fatigue in Sjögren syndrome with rituximab: results of a randomised, double-blind, placebo-controlled pilot study. Ann Rheum Dis 2008;67:1541–4.

9. Medawar PB. Immunological tolerance. Science 1961;133:303–6.

10. Gallucci S, Matzinger P. Danger signals: SOS to the immune system. Curr Opin Immunol 2001;13:114–9.

11. Medzhitov R, Janeway CA Jr. Decoding the patterns of self and nonself by the innate immune system. Science 2002;296:298–300.

12. Janeway CA Jr, Medzhitov R. Innate immune recognition. Annu Rev Immunol 2002;20:197–216.

13. Medzhitov R, Janeway C Jr. Innate immune recognition: mechanisms and pathways. Immunol Rev 2000;173:89–97.

14. Janeway CA Jr, Medzhitov R. Introduction: the role of innate immunity in the adaptive immune response. Semin Immunol 1998;10:349–50.

15. Morris G, Berk M, Walder K, et al. Central pathways causing fatigue in neuroinflammatory and autoimmune illnesses. BMC Med 2015;13:28.

16. Devauchelle-Pensec V, Mariette X, Jousse-Joulin S, et al. Treatment of primary Sjögren syndrome with rituximab a randomized trial. Ann Intern Med 2014;160:233–42.

17. Gottenberg J-E, Cinquetti G, Larroche C, et al. Efficacy of rituximab in systemic manifestations of primary Sjögren's syndrome: results in 78 patients of the Auto-Immune and Rituximab registry. Ann Rheum Dis 2013;72(6):1026–31.

18. Seror R, Sordet C, Guillevin L, et al. Tolerance and efficacy of rituximab and changes in serum B cell biomarkers in patients with systemic complications of primary Sjögren's syndrome. Ann Rheum Dis 2007;66(3):351–7.

19. Gottenberg JE, Guillevin L, Lambotte O, et al. Tolerance and short term efficacy of rituximab in 43 patients with systemic autoimmune diseases. Ann Rheum Dis 2005;64:913–20.

20. St Clair EW, Levesque MC, Prak ETL, et al. Rituximab therapy for primary Sjögren's syndrome: an open-label clinical trial and mechanistic analysis. Arthritis Rheum 2013;65:1097–106.

21. Meiners P, Vissink A, Kroese F, et al. Abatacept treatment reduces disease activity in early primary Sjögren's syndrome (open-label proof of concept ASAP study). Ann Rheum Dis 2014;73:1393–6.

22. Adler S, Körner M, Förger F, et al. Evaluation of histologic, serologic, and clinical changes in response to abatacept treatment of primary Sjögren's syndrome: a pilot study. Arthritis Care Res 2013;65:1862–8.

23. De Vita S, Quartuccio L, Seror R, et al. THU0392 efficacy and safety of belimumab given for 12 months in primary Sjögren's syndrome: the BELISS open-label Phase II study. Ann Rheum Dis 2015;74:338–9.

24. Mariette X, Seror R, Quartuccio L, et al. Efficacy and safety of belimumab in primary Sjögren's syndrome: results of the BELISS open-label phase II study. Ann Rheum Dis 2015;74(3):526–31.

25. Rasmussen A, Radfar L, Lewis D, et al. Previous diagnosis of Sjögren's Syndrome as rheumatoid arthritis or systemic lupus erythematosus. Rheumatology (Oxford) 2016. [pii:kew023; Epub ahead of print].

26. Davis LA, Goldstein B, Tran V, et al. Applying choosing wisely: antinuclear antibody (ANA) and sub-serology testing in a safety net hospital system. Open Rheumatol J 2015;9:82–7.

27. Metz LM, Seland TP, Fritzler MJ. An analysis of the frequency of Sjögren's syndrome in a population of multiple sclerosis patients. J Clin Lab Immunol 1989;30:121–5.

28. Fritzler MJ, Pauls JD, Kinsella TD, et al. Antinuclear, anticytoplasmic and anti-Sjögren's syndrome antigen A (SS-A/Ro) antibodies in female blood donors. Clin Immunol Immunopathol 1985;36:120–8.

29. David-Bajar KM, Bennion SD, DeSpain JD, et al. Clinical, histologic, and immuno-fluorescent distinctions between subacute cutaneous lupus erythematosus and discoid lupus erythematosus. J Invest Dermatol 1992;99:251–7.

30. Jonsson R, Gordon TP, Konttinen YT. Recent advances in understanding molecular mechanisms in the pathogenesis and antibody profile of Sjögren's syndrome. Curr Rheumatol Rep 2003;5:311–6.

31. Gordon TP, Bolstad AI, Rischmueller M, et al. Autoantibodies in primary Sjögren's syndrome: new insights into mechanisms of autoantibody diversification and disease pathogenesis. Autoimmunity 2001;34:123–32.

32. Tan EM, Smolen JS, McDougal JS, et al. A critical evaluation of enzyme immunoassays for detection of antinuclear autoantibodies of defined specificities. I. Precision, sensitivity, and specificity. Arthritis Rheum 1999;42:455–64.

33. Tan EM, Feltkamp TE, Smolen JS, et al. Range of antinuclear antibodies in "healthy" individuals. Arthritis Rheum 1997;40:1601–11.

34. Pottel H, Wiik A, Locht H, et al. Clinical optimization and multicenter validation of antigen-specific cut-off values on the INNO-LIA™ ANA Update for the detection of autoantibodies in connective tissue disorders. Clin Exp Rheumatol 2004;22:579–88.

35. De Bosschere K, Wiik A, Gordon T, et al. Clinical optimization and multicenter validation of antigen-specific cut-off values on the INNO-LIAr ANA Update for the detection of autoantibodies in connective tissue disorders. Arthritis Res 2002;4:1.

36. Cabot RC, Harris NL, Shepard J-AO, et al. Case 14-2011: A Woman with Asymmetric Sensory Loss and Paresthesias. N Engl J Med 2011;364:1856–65.

37. Baccala R, Welch MJ, Gonzalez-Quintial R, et al. Type I interferon is a therapeutic target for virus-induced lethal vascular damage. Proc Natl Acad Sci U S A 2014;111:8925–30.

38. Norheim KB, Jonsson G, Omdal R. Biological mechanisms of chronic fatigue. Rheumatology 2011;50:1009–18.

39. Morris G, Berk M, Galecki P, et al. The neuro-immune pathophysiology of central and peripheral fatigue in systemic immune-inflammatory and neuro-immune diseases. Mol Neurobiol 2016;53(2):1195–219.

40. Maes M. Inflammatory and oxidative and nitrosative stress pathways underpinning chronic fatigue, somatization and psychosomatic symptoms. Curr Opin Psychiatry 2009;22:75–83.

41. Chun J, Hartung HP. Mechanism of action of oral fingolimod (FTY720) in multiple sclerosis. Clin Neuropharmacol 2010;33:91.

42. Lucas K, Morris G, Anderson G, et al. The toll-like receptor radical cycle pathway: a new drug target in immune-related chronic fatigue. CNS Neurol Disord Drug Targets 2015;14(7):838–54.

43. Bårdsen K, Nilsen MM, Kvaløy JT, et al. Heat shock proteins and chronic fatigue in primary Sjögren's syndrome. Innate Immun 2016;22(3):162–7.

44. Isenberg DA, Merrill JT. Why, why, why de-lupus (does so badly in clinical trials). Expert Rev Clin Immunol 2016;12(2):95–8.

45. Stern ME, Beuerman RW, Fox RI, et al. A unified theory of the role of the ocular surface in dry eye. Adv Exp Med Biol 1998;438:643–51.

46. Stern ME, Beuerman RW, Fox RI, et al. The pathology of dry eye: the interaction between the ocular surface and lacrimal glands. Cornea 1998;17:584–9.

47. Turpie B, Yoshimura T, Gulati A, et al. Sjögren's syndrome-like ocular surface disease in thrombospondin-1 deficient mice. Am J Pathol 2009;175:1136–47.
48. Moulton EA, Becerra L, Rosenthal P, et al. An approach to localizing corneal pain representation in human primary somatosensory cortex. PLoS One 2012;7(9): e44643.
49. Daniels TE, Cox D, Shiboski CH, et al. Associations between salivary gland histopathologic diagnoses and phenotypic features of Sjögren's syndrome among 1,726 registry participants. Arthritis Rheum 2011;63:2021–30.
50. Theander E, Vasaitis L, Baecklund E, et al. Lymphoid organisation in labial salivary gland biopsies is a possible predictor for the development of malignant lymphoma in primary Sjögren's syndrome. Ann Rheum Dis 2011;70:1363–8.
51. Konttinen YT, Sorsa T, Hukkanen M, et al. Topology of innervation of labial salivary glands by protein gene product 9.5 and synaptophysin immunoreactive nerves in patients with Sjögren's syndrome. J Rheumatol 1992;19:30–7.
52. Pflugfelder SC, Solomon A, Stern ME. The diagnosis and management of dry eye: a twenty-five-year review. Cornea 2000;19:644–9.
53. Dartt DA. Neural regulation of lacrimal gland secretory processes: relevance in dry eye diseases. Prog Retin Eye Res 2009;28:155–77.

APPENDIX 1

The functional circuit in SS

Afferent signals from the periphery (mouth and eye) travel through defined pathways to the lacrimatory and salivatory nuclei of the cranial nerve V.[46,52]

Quiescent microglial cells become activated and release a series of factors that will modulate the neural transmissions transmitted to the cerebral cortex. These pathways and mediators have been elucidated in elegant murine model.[47,53]

Immune Signal Pathways in Midbrain (Targets for Sjögren's Syndrome)

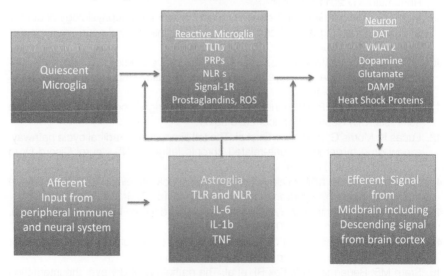

New Treatment Guidelines for Sjögren's Disease

Frederick B. Vivino, MD, MS[a],*, Steven E. Carsons, MD[b,c], Gary Foulks, MD[d], Troy E. Daniels, DDS, MS[e], Ann Parke, MD[f], Michael T. Brennan, DDS, MHS[g], S. Lance Forstot, MD[h], R. Hal Scofield, MD[i], Katherine M. Hammitt, MA[j]

KEYWORDS

- Sjögren's • Treatment • Caries • Fatigue • Dry eye • Arthritis • DMARDS
- Biologics

KEY POINTS

- Sjögren's disease (SD) is associated with a high burden of illness, poor quality of life, and increased health care costs.
- All SD patients with xerostomia should be given fluoride for caries prophylaxis.
- Proper treatment of dry eyes necessitates comprehensive assessment to determine severity level and the relative contributions of aqueous tear deficiency versus meibomian gland dysfunction.
- Disease-modifying antirheumatic drugs can be used to treat inflammatory musculoskeletal pain starting with hydroxychloroquine as first-line therapy.

Continued

Conflict of Interest Disclosures: Biogen (F.B. Vivino, S.E. Carson). Coda, Inc; Kala, Inc; Lexitas, Inc; Parion, Inc; Shire Pharmaceuticals, Inc; TearLab, Inc (G. Foulks). None (T.E. Daniels, K.M. Hammitt). UCB; Biogen (A. Parke). Daiichi Sankyo (M.T. Brennan). Alcon; Allergan; Bausch & Lomb; Eleven Biotherapeutics; Nicox; TearScience (S.L. Forstot). UCB (R.H. Scofield).
[a] Division of Rheumatology, Penn Presbyterian Medical Center, Penn Sjögren's Center, Penn Medicine University City, University of Pennsylvania, 3737 Market Street, Philadelphia, PA 19104, USA; [b] Division of Rheumatology, Allergy and Immunology, Winthrop University Hospital, 120 Mineola Boulevard, Suite 410, Mineola, NY 11501, USA; [c] Stony Brook University School of Medicine, Stony Brook, 120 Mineola Boulevard, Mineola, NY 11501, USA; [d] Department of Ophthalmology and Vision Science, University of Louisville School of Medicine, 301 East Muhammad Ali Boulevard, Louisville, KY 40202, USA; [e] Department of Orofacial Sciences, UCSF Schools of Dentistry and Medicine, 521 Parnassus Avenue, Clinic Sci, San Francisco, CA 94143, USA; [f] Division of Rheumatology, St. Francis Hospital & Medical Center, 114 Woodland Street, Hartford, CT 06105, USA; [g] Department of Oral Medicine, Carolinas Medical Center, 1000 Blythe Boulevard, Charlotte, NC 28203, USA; [h] Corneal Consultants of Colorado, 8381 Southpark Lane, Littleton, CO 80120, USA; [i] Department of Veterans Affairs, Oklahoma Medical Research Foundation, University of Oklahoma Health Sciences Center, 1000 North Lincoln Boulevard, #2900, Oklahoma City, OK 73104, USA; [j] Sjögren's Syndrome Foundation, 6707 Democracy Boulevard, Suite 325, Bethesda, MD 20817, USA
* Corresponding author.
E-mail address: frederick.vivino@uphs.upenn.edu

Rheum Dis Clin N Am 42 (2016) 531–551
http://dx.doi.org/10.1016/j.rdc.2016.03.010
0889-857X/16/$ – see front matter © 2016 Elsevier Inc. All rights reserved.

Continued

- Fatigue is most effectively managed with self-care measures and exercise.
- Biological therapy like rituximab is best used in SD patients with serious organ manifestations who fail more conservative treatments.

INTRODUCTION

Among all the chronic autoimmune rheumatic disorders, Sjögren's disease (SD) is among the most difficult to evaluate and manage. Clinicians are frequently challenged to differentiate symptoms related to disease activity from those that result from pre-existing damage. Additionally, the presence of multiple SD-related comorbidities, including anxiety, depression and fibromyalgia,[1,2] may influence the severity of patient symptoms and further complicate the evaluation process. Furthermore, in the clinical setting, a thorough investigation of patient complaints will often reveal multiple potential causes for the same symptom.[3]

Presently, no cure or remittive agent for SD exists. Treatment goals remain (1) symptom palliation, (2) prevention of complications and, (3) for rheumatologists, proper selection of patients for immunosuppressive therapy. In SD the frequent occurrence of oral and ocular manifestations and complications also mandates a multidisciplinary approach to optimize care. Unfortunately, the paucity of well-designed, controlled studies in the SD medical and dental literature frequently leaves the clinician with little guidance. Therefore, the approach to treating SD in the United States has differed widely among various institutions and providers.

HIGH BURDEN OF ILLNESS

Several studies have documented that quality of life (QOL) is diminished in primary SD subjects compared with healthy controls[1,4,5] and, in some cases, diminished to the degree seen in other subject groups, such as those with rheumatoid arthritis (RA) and/or fibromyalgia.[5] One study found less overall end organ damage in primary SD compared with systemic lupus (SLE) but concluded that the degree of functional disability was the same for both disorders.[6] Patients with SD may also incur increased health care costs[7,9] and, not surprisingly, increased dental care costs.[9] A study from England reported that annual health care costs in primary SD (£2188) were twice that of community controls (£949) and comparable to those of subjects with RA (£2693).[8] Thus, the burden of illness in primary SD is quite substantial.

GUIDELINES DEVELOPMENT

In 2010, the Sjögren's Syndrome Foundation (SSF) enlisted the help of more than 200 professional volunteers nationwide to develop the first ever clinical practice guidelines (CPGs) for SD patients in the United States. The framework for this process is summarized in **Fig. 1**. The goals were to improve the quality and consistency of care and to ease the uncertainty of providers, patients, and insurers regarding coverage and reimbursement issues. All working groups followed a highly rigorous process with guidance from major professional organizations including the Institute of Medicine, American Dental Association, American Academy of Ophthalmology (AAO), and the American College of Rheumatology (ACR). The Appraisal of Guidelines for Research and Evaluation (AGREE) was used.[10,11] Overreaching methodological principles

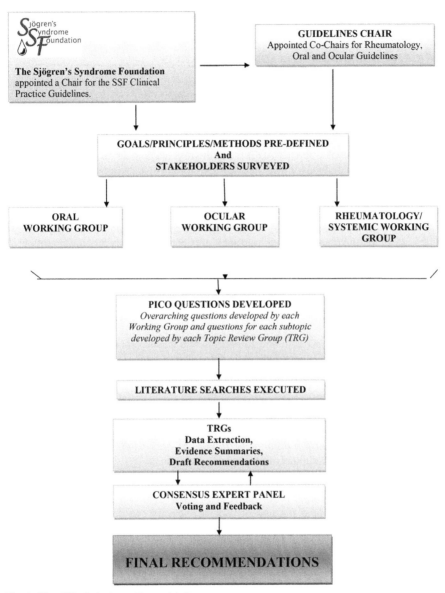

Fig. 1. The SSF clinical practice guidelines process.

included transparency, involvement of key stakeholders, and consistency of methods. All participants completed ACR conflict of interest forms.

DEFINING CLINICAL ISSUES

All key stakeholders, including patients and providers of various disciplines, from academia and the community, were surveyed to identify pertinent clinical issues. Topics were assigned to 1 of 3 working groups: Oral, Ocular, or Rheumatologic-Systemic; prioritized; and reformatted as PICO (population, intervention, comparison, and outcome) questions.[12] Bias was reduced as much as possible by defining a priori all methodology elements, including protocol worksheets, data extraction tables, and literature search terms.

TOPIC REVIEW AND THE DELPHI CONSENSUS PROCESS

Topic review groups (TRGs) of at least 2 to 3 providers were established for each clinical question to review the medical or dental literature, complete data extraction tables, and write an evidence summary. The TRG, as a whole, rated the strength of the evidence, developed a draft recommendation, and rated the strength of the recommendation based on a variation of grading of recommendations, assessment, development, and evaluation (GRADE).[13] For the dry eye guidelines the AAO Preferred Practice Pattern guidelines for level of evidence were also followed.[14] Any definition of primary SD (ie, SD without an associated connective tissue disorder) based on published classification criteria were accepted for guideline development. Data on patients with secondary SD were not used in this analysis.

A consensus expert panel (CEP) of pertinent specialists, providers from other disciplines, and stakeholders provided feedback and voted on each recommendation. A modified Delphi process was used with 75% agreement required for consensus. Revision of guidelines that failed to achieve consensus was permitted up to 3 rounds before the recommendation was discarded.

Guidelines for Oral Management

Rationale
Salivary dysfunction in SD can lead to serious and costly oral health complications. Study subjects with SD have significantly more dental caries, tooth extractions, and higher lifetime dental costs then do controls.[15] SD patients who lose their dentition often have problems with denture wear and find that dental implants provide the only viable long-term alternative. Most patients in the United States lack sufficient dental insurance to cover these expenses and pay most costs out-of-pocket. It is, therefore, incumbent on every dentist and oral medicine specialist to consider the diagnosis of SD in patients with accelerated caries and initiate a management program for caries prophylaxis early in the disease course.

Recommendations
To develop CPGs for caries prophylaxis in SD, the Oral Working Group reviewed dental literature concerning the use of fluoride, salivary stimulation, antimicrobials, and remineralizing agents. **Fig. 2** is a summary of this process. Further details, including findings from extensive literature reviews, protocol worksheets, data extraction tables, and summaries of dental evidence, have been previously reported.[16] The clinical questions and oral guidelines for caries prophylaxis in SD are summarized in **Box 1**. The clinician is encouraged to consider all recommendations as potential therapies to be used either singly or in combination for the individual patient.

Guidelines for Ocular Management

Rationale
At least 2 prior surveys of SD patients conducted by the SSF have documented dry eye to be the single most troublesome symptom in SD.[17,18] Additionally, dry eye is recognized as a debilitating symptom in the US Social Security Administration Disability Guidelines, which included SD as a specific listing for the first time in 2006. Dry eye can seriously compromise QOL[19] and at least 1 study suggested that the impact of dry eye on QOL was comparable to that seen in patients with moderate to severe angina.[20]

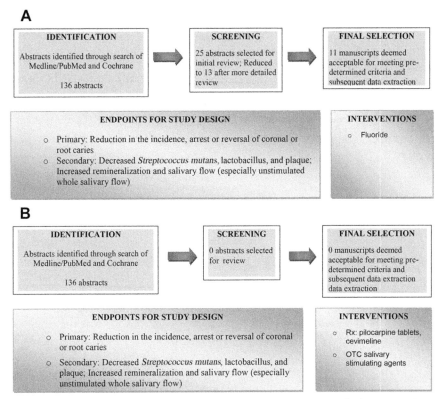

A

IDENTIFICATION	SCREENING	FINAL SELECTION
Abstracts identified through search of Medline/PubMed and Cochrane 136 abstracts	25 abstracts selected for initial review; Reduced to 13 after more detailed review	11 manuscripts deemed acceptable for meeting pre-determined criteria and subsequent data extraction

ENDPOINTS FOR STUDY DESIGN

- o Primary: Reduction in the incidence, arrest or reversal of coronal or root caries
- o Secondary: Decreased *Streptococcus mutans*, lactobacillus, and plaque; Increased remineralization and salivary flow (especially unstimulated whole salivary flow)

INTERVENTIONS

- o Fluoride

B

IDENTIFICATION	SCREENING	FINAL SELECTION
Abstracts identified through search of Medline/PubMed and Cochrane 136 abstracts	0 abstracts selected for review	0 manuscripts deemed acceptable for meeting pre-determined criteria and subsequent data extraction data extraction

ENDPOINTS FOR STUDY DESIGN

- o Primary: Reduction in the incidence, arrest or reversal of coronal or root caries
- o Secondary: Decreased *Streptococcus mutans*, lactobacillus, and plaque; Increased remineralization and salivary flow (especially unstimulated whole salivary flow)

INTERVENTIONS

- o Rx: pilocarpine tablets, cevimeline
- o OTC salivary stimulating agents

Fig. 2. (*A*) Review of fluoride use for caries prevention in SD. (*B*) Review of salivary stimulation for caries prevention in SD. OTC, over-the-counter. (*C*) Review of antimicrobials for caries prevention in SD. (*D*) Review of nonfluoride remineralizing agents for caries prevention in SD.

Terminology

The development of ocular guidelines for the evaluation and management of dry eyes for SD used the definition of dry eye and other terminology reported in the 2007 International Dry Eye Workshop (DEWS).[21] The DEWS report defined terms to characterize patient subsets, as well as clinical issues, and defined dry eye as, "a multi-factorial disease of the tears and ocular surface that results in symptoms of discomfort, visual disturbance, and tear film instability with potential damage to the ocular surface. It is accompanied by increased osmolarity of the tear film and inflammation of the ocular surface."

Dry eye is classified into 2 categories: (1) aqueous-deficient dry eye related to decreased tear production and (2) evaporative dry eye most commonly caused by meibomian gland dysfunction (blepharitis). Both types of dry eye may occur in SD and often coexist in the same individual. Most patients are symptomatic and describe their discomfort as burning, stinging, foreign body sensation (grittiness), itching, or pain. Symptoms of visual disturbance may include fluctuation or blurring of vision, especially during reading or computer work, with transient improvement after blinking or the instillation of artificial tears. Interestingly, a recent study reported that as many as 40% of SD subjects with clear objective evidence of dry eyes had no symptoms, thus underscoring the necessity to thoroughly evaluate all SD patients for dry eye regardless of symptoms.[22]

Evaluation

The Ocular Working Group stressed the importance of comprehensive assessment of the SD patient to determine the cause and severity of dry eye before recommending

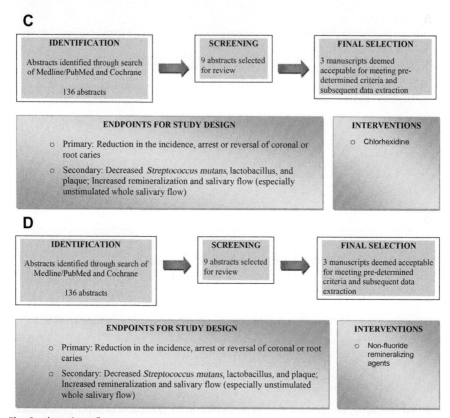

C

IDENTIFICATION	SCREENING	FINAL SELECTION
Abstracts identified through search of Medline/PubMed and Cochrane 136 abstracts	9 abstracts selected for review	3 manuscripts deemed acceptable for meeting pre-determined criteria and subsequent data extraction

ENDPOINTS FOR STUDY DESIGN	INTERVENTIONS
o Primary: Reduction in the incidence, arrest or reversal of coronal or root caries o Secondary: Decreased *Streptococcus mutans*, lactobacillus, and plaque; Increased remineralization and salivary flow (especially unstimulated whole salivary flow)	o Chlorhexidine

D

IDENTIFICATION	SCREENING	FINAL SELECTION
Abstracts identified through search of Medline/PubMed and Cochrane 136 abstracts	9 abstracts selected for review	3 manuscripts deemed acceptable for meeting pre-determined criteria and subsequent data extraction

ENDPOINTS FOR STUDY DESIGN	INTERVENTIONS
o Primary: Reduction in the incidence, arrest or reversal of coronal or root caries o Secondary: Decreased *Streptococcus mutans*, lactobacillus, and plaque; Increased remineralization and salivary flow (especially unstimulated whole salivary flow)	o Non-fluoride remineralizing agents

Fig. 2. (*continued*)

treatment. This process involves the assessment of key ocular symptoms as described previously, as well as the examination of several objective parameters, including tear production, tear film stability, tear osmolarity, lid margin disease, and ocular surface damage. A summary of the diagnostic evaluation and recommended order of tests is included in **Table 1**.

Recommendations

To develop SD-specific ocular CPGs, the dry eye literature was reviewed according to preselected criteria as summarized in **Fig. 3**. Studies on non-SD dry eye disease also guided management whenever considered essential. The CPGs for dry eye management in SD are outlined in **Table 2** and organized by type of dry eye disease (aqueous deficient vs meibomian gland dysfunction) and level of severity. The latter is determined mainly by the presence or absence of ocular surface staining and the staining pattern. Conjunctival staining usually occurs before corneal staining and medial staining often occurs before temporal conjunctival staining. Early corneal staining is most often observed in the inferonasal cornea with central staining occurring later. A classic pattern of interpalpebral staining across the medial conjunctiva, cornea, and temporal conjunctiva, or the presence of ocular filaments, indicates advanced dry eye disease. If the results of treatment of the SD patient at a given level of severity are insufficient, the eye care provider is encouraged to follow recommendations for the next level of severity.

A detailed description of therapeutic options and the evidence that supports these recommendations has been previously reported.[23] Patient education regarding the nature of the problem, aggravating factors and treatment goals is essential to

---

Box 1
Oral management guidelines for caries prophylaxis

Use of fluoride
Clinical questions

- In primary SD patients, does the use of a topical fluoride compared with no topical fluoride reduce the incidence, arrest, or reverse coronal or root caries?
- In primary SD patients, is one topical fluoride agent more effective than another in reducing the incidence, or to arrest or reverse, coronal or root caries?

Recommendation

Topical fluoride should be used in SD patients with dry mouth.

No information was available to answer the second question.

Strength of recommendation: strong

Salivary stimulation
Clinical questions

- In primary SD patients, does salivary stimulation compared with not stimulating saliva flow reduce the incidence, arrest, or reverse coronal or root caries?

Recommendation

While no studies to date link improved salivary function in SS patients to caries prevention, it is generally understood in the oral health community that increasing saliva may contribute to decreased caries incidence. Based on its expert opinion, the TRG recommends that SD patients with dry mouth increase saliva through gustatory, masticatory stimulation, and pharmaceutical agents; for example, sugar-free lozenges and/or chewing gum, xylitol, mannitol, and the prescription medications pilocarpine and cevimeline.

Strength of recommendation: weak

Antimicrobials
Clinical questions

- In primary SD patients, does the use of antimicrobial agents compared with placebo reduce the incidence, arrest, or reverse coronal or root caries?

Recommendation

Chlorhexidine administered by varnish, gel, or rinse may be considered in SD patients with dry mouth and a high root caries rate.

Strength of recommendation: weak

Nonfluoride remineralizing agents
Clinical questions

- In primary SD patients, does the use of nonfluoride remineralization agents compared with placebo reduce the incidence, arrest, or reverse coronal or root caries?
- In primary SD patients, does the use of nonfluoride remineralization agents compared with the use of fluoride reduce the incidence, arrest, or reverse coronal or root caries?

Recommendation

Nonfluoride remineralizing agents may be considered as an adjunct therapy in SD patients with dry mouth and a high root caries rate.

Insufficient information was available to answer the second question.

Strength of recommendation: moderate

Table 1
Evaluation of dry eye

Observation or Test	What is Examined	Tools	Sign of Dry Eye
1. Direct Observation	Tear function, tear stability and ocular surface	Corneal light reflex biomicroscope (additional instruments are available in the research setting)	Tear film instability Ocular surface irregularity
	Meibomian gland disease	Biomicroscope	Presence of foamy debris
2. Osmolarity	Tear composition: levels of inflammatory mediators in tear film and conjunctiva	Osmometer (mostly limited to research settings but units are increasingly available for clinical practice)	Elevated osmolarity of the tear film
3. Fluorescein Tear Break-Up Time	Tear film stability	Fluorescein dye Slit-lamp	Rapid tear film breakup (<10 s)
4. Corneal Staining	Ocular surface evaluation	Fluorescein Rose bengal or lissamine green dye	Staining observed of mucus strands, filaments, and unprotected areas of the epithelium Staining patterns can designate severity of dry eye
5. Schirmer 1 Test or Phenol Red Thread Test	Tear secretion rate	Schirmer tear test strip Small thread impregnated with phenol red dye A fluorophotometer is more sensitive than either of these but is usually not available in the clinical setting	Schirmer 1: <5–7 mm of wetting after 5 min Phenol red thread test: <10 mm of wetting after 15 s

successful management. Strategies include use of topical tear substitutes, gels and ointments, anti-inflammatory therapies, secretagogues, punctal occlusion, autologous serum tears, mucolytic agents, therapeutic contact lenses, and management of eyelid disease.

Guidelines for Rheumatologic-Systemic Management

Rationale

Morbidity in SD results not only from untreated sicca but also from internal organ involvement (**Table 3**) and an increased incidence of non-Hodgkin B cell lymphomas.[24] The current treatment algorithms for serious organ manifestations of SD are frequently borrowed from management strategies used for closely related disorders such as SLE and RA. Initially, 97 potential topics for guideline development were identified by review of stakeholder surveys. After further discussion, the list was narrowed to 16 topics that were ranked by vote of the Rheumatologic-Systemic Working Group. Initial efforts were focused on the 3 most important topic

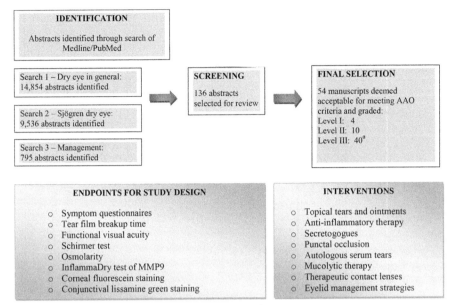

Fig. 3. Review of treatments for dry eye. [a] Best evidence.

areas: treatment of inflammatory musculoskeletal pain, management of fatigue, and the use of biological medications in SD. Study selection criteria and results of literature review for the first 3 topics are summarized in **Fig. 4**. Carsons and colleagues[25] provide further details, including findings from extensive literature reviews, protocol worksheets, data extraction tables, evidence summaries, and discussion of the recommendations.

Use of disease-modifying antirheumatic drugs for inflammatory musculoskeletal pain

Inflammatory arthralgias, myalgias and, in some cases, synovitis, can occur in SD and contribute to disease morbidity and patient disability. Guidelines for the use of disease-modifying antirheumatic drugs (DMARDS) for treatment of inflammatory musculoskeletal pain are represented in **Box 2** and use a stepwise approach with hydroxychloroquine (HCQ) listed as first-line therapy. Although a recent randomized controlled study of HCQ in SD failed to meet the primary endpoint for pain,[26] the moderate strength of the recommendation and 92% agreement of the CEP as guided by the modified Delphi process is based on the significant reported improvement of inflammatory markers and musculoskeletal pain in other studies,[27–30] a moderate level of confidence that the guideline recommendation reflected best clinical practice and that sufficient evidence existed that potential benefits exceeded potential harms. In instances in which therapies were deemed equivalent with similar safety profiles, recommendations were grouped together to allow the physician final choice based on clinical experience and patient profile.

Methotrexate (MTX) was determined to be second-line therapy after HCQ based on some evidence for a true net effect[30,31] and moderate confidence regarding a good safety profile. Although there is no reported evidence to support this guideline, combined therapy with HCQ and MTX was recommended as the third step if either drug alone was ineffective. This statement was based on the collective experience of the TRG-CEP and the knowledge that both therapies have been successfully combined

Table 2
Guidelines for management of dry eye based on cause and severity

Diagnosis	Treatment | Severity Level 1[a]	Severity Level 2	Severity Level 3	Severity Level 4	Evidence[b]	Recommendation[c]
Dry eye disease: aqueous deficiency without meibomian gland disease	Education and environment or diet modification	—	—	—	Good	Strong
	Elimination of offending systemic medication				Good	Strong
	Artificial tears, gels, ointments				Good	Strong
	—	Omega 3 essential fatty acid supplement	—	—	Moderate	Moderate
		Anti-inflammatory therapy: cyclosporine			Good	Moderate
		Anti-inflammatory therapy: pulse steroids			Good	Moderate
		Punctal plugs			Good	Moderate
		Secretagogues			Good	Moderate
		Moisture chamber spectacles			Good	Moderate
	—	—	Topical autologous serum	—	Good	Moderate
			Contact lenses		Good	Moderate
			Permanent punctal occlusion		Good	Moderate
	—	—	—	Systemic anti-inflammatory medication	Moderate	Weak
				Eyelid surgery	Good	Moderate

		Evidence[b]	Recommendation[c]
Dry eye disease: aqueous deficiency with meibomian gland disease	Education and environment or diet modification	—	Good	Strong
	Elimination of offending systemic medication		Good	Strong
	Artificial tears with lipid component		Good	Strong
	Eyelid therapy: warm compress, massage		Good	Strong
	Omega 3 essential fatty acid supplement	—	Moderate	Moderate
	Anti-inflammatory therapy: cyclosporine		Good	Moderate
	Anti-inflammatory therapy: topical steroids		Good	Moderate
	Topical azithromycin		Good	Moderate
	Liposomal spray		Good	Moderate
	Possible oral doxycycline		Good	Moderate
	Expression of meibomian glands		Good	Moderate
	Punctal plugs		Good	Moderate
	Secretagogues		Good	Moderate
	Moisture chamber spectacles		Good	Moderate
	Topical autologous serum	—	Good	Moderate
	Contact lenses		Good	Moderate
	Permanent punctal occlusion		Good	Moderate
	LipiFlow pulsed thermal compression		Insufficient	Weak
	Probing of meibomian gland	—	Insufficient	Weak
	Systemic anti-inflammatory medication		Moderate	Weak
	Eyelid surgery		Good	Moderate

[a] Assumes use of the International DEWS severity scale.
[b] Evidence is graded as good, moderate, and insufficient.
[c] Recommendations are strong, moderate, and weak.

Table 3
Extraoral and extraglandular manifestations of Sjögren's disease

Area Affected	Symptoms
General	Fatigue, malaise, fevers
Ear, nose, and throat	Epistaxis, otitis media, conduction deafness, recurrent sinusitis
Gastrointestinal	Esophageal dysmotility, esophageal webs, reflux, atrophic gastritis, autoimmune pancreatitis, liver disease
Genitourinary	Vaginitis sicca, interstitial cystitis
Hematologic	Anemia, leukopenia, lymphopenia, cryoglobulinemia, lymphoma
Lungs	Xerotrachea, recurrent bronchitis or pneumonia, interstitial pneumonitis, pulmonary fibrosis, lung nodules, bronchiectasis, bronchiolitis obliterans with organizing pneumonia
Neurologic	Peripheral neuropathy, cranial neuropathy, autonomic neuropathy, central nervous system involvement
Renal	Interstitial nephritis, hyposthenuria, renal tubular acidosis (Types I, II), glomerulonephritis (rare)
Rheumatologic	Arthralgias, polyarthritis, myalgias, myositis, Raynaud's phenomenon
Skin	Xeroderma, purpura, urticaria, vasculitis

to treat arthritis in closely related autoimmune rheumatic disorders (eg, RA, SLE). When adding MTX to HCQ, physicians may choose to lower the dose of HCQ as maintenance therapy.

Although no formal studies have reported efficacy on the short-term ($\leq$1 month) use of corticosteroids ($\leq$15 mg/day) for inflammatory musculoskeletal pain in SD, this practice is frequently followed in the United States and, therefore, listed as fourth-line therapy when the first 3 treatment approaches fail. There was a strong level of agreement among the CEP that this treatment approach reflects best clinical practice. Longer-term use of corticosteroids at similar doses was deemed equally efficacious but the strength of recommendation was lowered to moderate due to concern over potential side effects. Although this task can be quite challenging, the CEP recommended that every possible effort be made to find a steroid-sparing agent as soon as possible in glucocorticoid-responsive SD patients.

The algorithm concluded with grouping of leflunomide, sulfasalazine, and azathioprine together, followed by listing cyclosporine as a potential therapy for inflammatory musculoskeletal pain in SD. Evidence for these recommendations is scant[32,33] and clinical experience with these medications in SD limited. One exception was emphasized. In situations when the SD patient has significant extraglandular involvement in association with inflammatory musculoskeletal pain, azathioprine would be preferred because of anecdotal evidence, case reports, and case series suggesting benefit for SD manifestations, including central nervous system disease, peripheral neuropathies, interstitial lung disease, and leukocytoclastic vasculitis.

Management of fatigue

Treatment of fatigue is among the greatest therapeutic challenges in the management of SD.[34] In guidelines development, the TRG-CEP emphasized that causes of fatigue in SS are numerous[3] and that proper therapy necessitates a thoughtful and comprehensive diagnostic approach. Guideline recommendations for fatigue are summarized in **Box 3**.

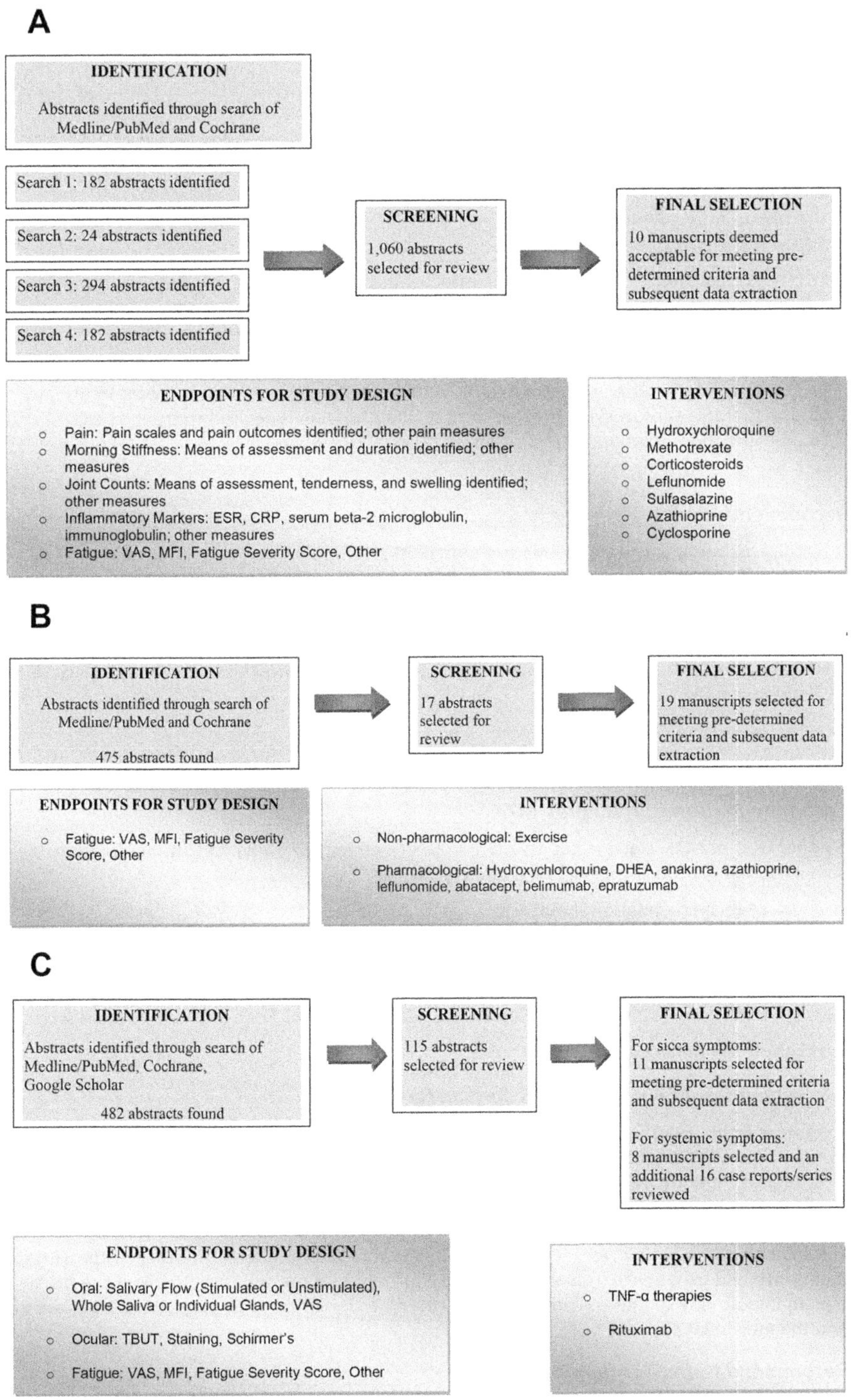

A

IDENTIFICATION

Abstracts identified through search of
Medline/PubMed and Cochrane

Search 1: 182 abstracts identified

Search 2: 24 abstracts identified

Search 3: 294 abstracts identified

Search 4: 182 abstracts identified

SCREENING

1,060 abstracts
selected for review

FINAL SELECTION

10 manuscripts deemed
acceptable for meeting pre-
determined criteria and
subsequent data extraction

ENDPOINTS FOR STUDY DESIGN

- Pain: Pain scales and pain outcomes identified; other pain measures
- Morning Stiffness: Means of assessment and duration identified; other measures
- Joint Counts: Means of assessment, tenderness, and swelling identified; other measures
- Inflammatory Markers: ESR, CRP, serum beta-2 microglobulin, immunoglobulin; other measures
- Fatigue: VAS, MFI, Fatigue Severity Score, Other

INTERVENTIONS

- Hydroxychloroquine
- Methotrexate
- Corticosteroids
- Leflunomide
- Sulfasalazine
- Azathioprine
- Cyclosporine

B

IDENTIFICATION

Abstracts identified through search of
Medline/PubMed and Cochrane

475 abstracts found

SCREENING

17 abstracts
selected for
review

FINAL SELECTION

19 manuscripts selected for
meeting pre-determined
criteria and subsequent data
extraction

ENDPOINTS FOR STUDY DESIGN

- Fatigue: VAS, MFI, Fatigue Severity Score, Other

INTERVENTIONS

- Non-pharmacological: Exercise

- Pharmacological: Hydroxychloroquine, DHEA, anakinra, azathioprine, leflunomide, abatacept, belimumab, epratuzumab

C

IDENTIFICATION

Abstracts identified through search of
Medline/PubMed, Cochrane,
Google Scholar

482 abstracts found

SCREENING

115 abstracts
selected for review

FINAL SELECTION

For sicca symptoms:
11 manuscripts selected for
meeting pre-determined criteria
and subsequent data extraction

For systemic symptoms:
8 manuscripts selected and an
additional 16 case reports/series
reviewed

ENDPOINTS FOR STUDY DESIGN

- Oral: Salivary Flow (Stimulated or Unstimulated), Whole Saliva or Individual Glands, VAS

- Ocular: TBUT, Staining, Schirmer's

- Fatigue: VAS, MFI, Fatigue Severity Score, Other

INTERVENTIONS

- TNF-α therapies

- Rituximab

Fig. 4. (*A*) Review of disease-modifying antirheumatic drug (DMARD) use for musculoskel-etal pain in SD. (*B*) Review of treatments for fatigue in SD. (*C*) Review of biological medica-tion use in SD.

Box 2
Guidelines for disease-modifying antirheumatic drug use for musculoskeletal pain in Sjögren's disease

DMARDs FOR INFLAMMATORY MSK PAIN

Recommendations are provided with the following caveats and then listed in a step-by-step process:

- The physician is advised to consider an individual patient's circumstances when weighing risks and benefits of each therapy.

- Insufficient evidence exists on the effectiveness of DMARDs in the treatment of inflammatory musculoskeletal pain in primary SD. However, recommendations will be formulated based on expert opinion as guided by the consensus group process.

- The following recommendations are listed in order of the Inflammatory Musculoskeletal TRG's preference for use in the treatment of inflammatory musculoskeletal pain in primary SD; if a therapy is insufficient in effectiveness, the physician is advised to try the next recommendation in sequence and so on.

Recommendation 1: Hydroxychloroquine (HCQ)

A first-line of treatment of inflammatory musculoskeletal pain in primary SD should be HCQ.

Strength of recommendation: moderate

Recommendation 2: Methotrexate (MTX)

If HCQ is not effective in the treatment of inflammatory musculoskeletal pain in primary SD, MTX alone may be considered.

Strength of recommendation: moderate

or

Recommendation 3: HCQ plus MTX

If either HCQ or MTX alone is not effective in the treatment of inflammatory musculoskeletal pain in primary SD, HCQ plus MTX may be considered.

Strength of recommendation: moderate

Recommendation 4a: Short-term corticosteroids

If HCQ plus MTX is not effective in the treatment of inflammatory musculoskeletal pain in primary SD, short term (1 month or less) corticosteroids of 15 mg or less a day may be considered.

Strength of recommendation: strong

Recommendation 4b: Long-term corticosteroids

Long-term (more than 1 month) 15 mg or less a day corticosteroids may be useful in the management of inflammatory musculoskeletal pain in primary SD but efforts should be made to find a steroid-sparing agent as soon as possible.

Strength of recommendation: moderate

The following 3 (5, 6, and 7a and 7b) recommendations are numbered in order of the TRG's preference and experience. However, the TRG is grouping these together to allow the physician to choose any of the following and in any order based on that physician's experience and the individual patient.

Recommendation 5: Leflunomide

If HCQ and/or MTX or short-term (1 month or less) corticosteroids are not effective in the treatment of inflammatory musculoskeletal pain in primary SD, leflunomide may be considered.

Strength of recommendation: weak

Recommendation 6: Sulfasalazine

If HCQ and/or MTX, corticosteroids, or leflunomide (Arava) are not effective in the treatment of inflammatory musculoskeletal pain in primary SD, sulfasalazine may be considered.

Strength of recommendation: weak

Recommendation 7a: Azathioprine

If HCQ and/or MTX, corticosteroids, leflunomide, or sulfasalazine are not effective in the treatment of inflammatory musculoskeletal pain in primary SD, azathioprine may be considered.

Strength of recommendation: weak

Recommendation 7b: Potential change in order

If major organ involvement occurs in the primary SD patient, azathioprine may be a better choice than leflunomide or sulfasalazine for the treatment of all complications, including inflammatory musculoskeletal pain.

Strength of recommendation: moderate

Recommendation 8: Cyclosporine

If HCQ and/or MTX, corticosteroids, leflunomide, azathioprine, or sulfasalazine are not effective in the treatment of inflammatory musculoskeletal pain in primary SD, cyclosporine may be considered.

Strength of recommendation: weak

The only strongly recommended treatment of fatigue in SD was exercise, which provides the same benefit for SD patients[35] that is seen in patients with RA, SLE, or multiple sclerosis. The panel also recommended that "hydroxychloroquine may be considered in selected situations to treat fatigue in Sjögren's." This approach is mainly based on uncontrolled studies as well as clinical experience and a favorable safety profile in both lupus and SD, given that evidence of benefit in placebo-controlled trials is lacking. Nevertheless, comments from the CEP during the first 2 voting rounds demonstrated strong support for keeping this option, especially in light of the perceived limitations of the controlled trials. When the draft recommendation was revised from "HCQ should not be used for fatigue" to the current recommendation listed previously, consensus agreement increased by 30% and enabled inclusion of this recommendation in the final guidelines. Currently, the CEP recommend against the use of dehydroepiandrosterone (DHEA)[36,37] and tumor necrosis factor (TNF)-α inhibitors[38,39] for fatigue, and found insufficient data and/or existing clinical experience to recommend use of anakinra, abatacept, belimumab, or epratuzumab for this indication.

Use of biologics in Sjögren's disease

Recently, the study of biological therapies as potential remittive agents for SD has generated tremendous interest in the SD community. CPGs for use of biologics in SD are summarized in **Box 4**. The CEP recommended against the use of TNF-α inhibitors in SD, based on findings from 2 earlier studies,[38,39] but emphasized this recommendation does not preclude the use of these agents in SD patients if needed for other indications (eg, overlapping manifestations with RA). The committee concluded that, among the various biologics studied to date, some evidence exists to justify the use of rituximab for sicca manifestations in selected patients with SD who otherwise fail more conservative and less costly measures. Although a recent, randomized, placebo-controlled trial of rituximab in SD failed to meet primary endpoints that included sicca symptoms,[40] an analysis of secondary outcome measures[41] and a

---

Box 3
Guidelines for treatment of fatigue in Sjögren's disease

Fatigue
Recommendation 1: Exercise

Education about self-care measures should include advice about exercise to reduce fatigue in SD.

Strength of recommendation: strong

Recommendation 2: Dehydroepiandrosterone (DHEA)

DHEA is not recommended for treatment of fatigue in SD.

Strength of recommendation: strong

Recommendation 3: HCQ

HCQ may be considered in selected situations to treat fatigue in SD.

Strength of recommendation: weak

Recommendation 4: Tumor necrosis factor (TNF)-α inhibitors

Neither etanercept nor infliximab is recommended for treatment of fatigue in SD.

Strength of recommendation: strong

For the following 10 therapeutic options addressed by the Fatigue TRG, there was insufficient evidence to issue a recommendation:

- Interleukin-1 inhibition (anakinra)
- Azathioprine
- Mycophenolate
- Zidovudine
- Doxycycline
- Lamivudine
- Leflunomide
- Abatacept
- Belimumab
- Epratuzumab

---

smaller randomized, placebo-controlled trial[42] provide evidence to support this recommendation. Rituximab was also recommended for SD patients with serious organ manifestations who fail more conservative and less costly therapies. This was based on results of a nonrandomized comparator trial[43] and other large studies that described outcomes for systemic or internal organ manifestations in SD patients.[44–47] Although not common, significant toxicity can be seen with rituximab as seen with other biologics. Patients with SD require careful monitoring for side effects as outlined in recommendation 6.

DISCUSSION AND FUTURE DIRECTIONS

SD remains a highly prevalent chronic autoimmune rheumatic disease with many unmet clinical needs. The process of CPG development has helped define the goals for

Box 4
Guidelines for use of biological medications in Sjögren's disease

Biological Therapies
Recommendation 1: TNF-α inhibitors

TNF-α inhibitors should not be used to treat sicca symptoms in patients with primary SD.

Strength of recommendation: strong

Recommendation 2: TNF-α inhibitor cautions

If TNF-α inhibition therapy is used for RA or other related overlap conditions in SD patients, health care providers should consider and monitor for the following:

- Lymphoma and other malignancies; health care providers should be cognizant that patients with primary SD have an increased risk of non-Hodgkin lymphoma compared with the general population
- Serious infections, including tuberculosis
- Invasive fungal infections
- Hepatitis B reactivation
- Hepatotoxicity
- Heart failure
- Cytopenias
- Hypersensitivity, serious infusion reactions
- Demyelinating disease

Strength of recommendation: strong

Recommendation 3: Rituximab for keratoconjunctivitis sicca (KCS)

Rituximab may be considered as a therapeutic option for KCS in patients with primary SD and for whom conventional therapies, including topical moisturizers, secretagogues, anti-inflammatories, immunomodulators, and punctual occlusion, have proven insufficient.

Strength of recommendation: weak

Recommendation 4: Rituximab for xerostomia

Rituximab may be considered as a therapeutic option for xerostomia in patients with primary SD with some evidence of residual salivary production, significant evidence of oral damage as determined by the clinician, and for whom conventional therapies, including topical moisturizers and secretagogues, have proven insufficient.

Strength of recommendation: weak

Recommendation 5: Rituximab for systemic symptoms

Rituximab may be considered as a therapeutic option for adults with primary SD and any or all of the following systemic manifestations:

- Cryoglobulinemia associated with vasculitis
- Vasculitis
- Severe parotid swelling
- Inflammatory arthritis
- Pulmonary disease
- Peripheral neuropathy, especially mononeuritis

Strength of recommendation: moderate

Recommendation 6: Rituximab cautions

Patients and health care providers should be aware that, although uncommon, significant harms may be associated with the use of rituximab and should exercise caution and observe for the following when using rituximab in SD patients:

- Infusion reactions
- Tumor lysis syndrome in patients with non-Hodgkin lymphoma
- Progressive multifocal leukoencephalopathy
- Hepatitis B reactivation with possible fulminant hepatitis
- Severe mucocutaneous reactions
- Infections
- Bowel obstruction and perforation
- Cardiac arrhythmias and angina
- Cytopenias
- Serious bacterial, viral, or fungal infections
- In pregnancy and nursing, the risk vs benefit must be carefully considered
- Health care providers should avoid giving live vaccines when patients are on rituximab.

Strength of recommendation: strong

---

future therapeutic studies. Of paramount importance is the need to develop SD-specific outcome measures that encompass the spectrum of organ system involvement and are sensitive to clinically meaningful change. Better staging to identify patients with early disease, and the discovery of novel biomarkers and/or genetic profiling to define specific patient subsets should facilitate better patient selection for targeted therapies. The design of future studies (eg, rituximab) should include evaluation time points and dosing regimens relevant to patients with SD rather than those with related disorders such as RA.

The working groups further recommended future clinical trials to (1) identify the most efficacious oral DMARD for inflammatory musculoskeletal pain; (2) expand studies of anti-B cell, anticytokine therapy (eg, BAFF, interleukin-6, interferon), inhibition of T-cell stimulation, and Janus kinase inhibitors for SD patients with early sicca and/or serious extraglandular manifestations; and (3) develop a multimodality approach for the management of SD-related fatigue, including pharmacologic and nonpharmacologic therapies.

Further research on the pathophysiology of dry eye as addressed in the recent second International DEWS will suggest new therapeutic targets for SD, including focused anti-inflammatory therapy (eg, topical anticytokines, integrin-directed therapy) and research into nanotechnology as applied to drug delivery for dry eye. Finally, further work in dentistry is needed to optimize the use of fluoride (eg, preparation, application, dosing regimen) and other adjunctive measures previously described for caries prevention in SD.

Guidelines will be revised as new information becomes available.

REFERENCES

1. Valtýsdóttir ST, Gudbjörnsson B, Lindqvist U, et al. Anxiety and depression in patients with primary Sjögren's syndrome. J Rheumatol 2000;27(1):165–9.

2. Vitali C, Tavoni A, Neri R, et al. Fibromyalgia Features in Patients with Primary Sjögren's Syndrome: Evidence of a Relationship with Psychological Depression. Scand J Rheumatol 1989;18(1):21–7.
3. Mishra R, Vivino FB. Diagnosis and management of fatigue. In: Wallace DJ, editor. The Sjögren's book. New York: The Sjögren's Syndrome Foundation and Oxford University Press; 2012. p. 228–34.
4. Segal B, Bowman SJ, Fox PC, et al. Primary Sjögren's Syndrome: health experiences and predictors of health quality among patients in the United States. Health Qual Life Outcomes 2009;7:46.
5. Strömbeck B, Ekdahl C, Manthorpe R, et al. Health-related quality of life in primary Sjögren's syndrome, rheumatoid arthritis and fibromyalgia compared to normal population data using SF-36. Scand J Rheumatol 2000;29(1):20–281.
6. Sutcliffe N, Stoll T, Pyke S, et al. Functional disability and end organ damage in patients with systemic lupus erythematosus (SLE), SLE and Sjögren's syndrome (SS) and primary SS. J Rheumatol 1998;25(1):63–8.
7. Bowman SJ, St Pierre Y, Sutcliffe N, et al. Estimating indirect costs in primary Sjögren's syndrome. J Rheumatol 2010;37(5):1010–5.
8. Callaghan R, Prabu A, Allan RB, et al, UK Sjögren's Interest Group. Direct healthcare costs and predictors of costs in patients with primary Sjögren's syndrome. Rheumatology (Oxford) 2007;46(1):105–11.
9. Fox PC, Bowman SJ, Segal B, et al. Oral involvement in primary Sjögren's syndrome. J Am Dent Assoc 2008;139(12):1592–601.
10. AGREE Collaboration. Development and validation of an international appraisal instrument for assessing the quality of clinical practice guidelines: the AGREE project. Qual Saf Health Care 2003;12(1):18–23.
11. AGREE Research Trust. Appraisal of guidelines for research and evaluation II. 2013. Available at: http://www.agreetrust.org/wp-content/uploads/2013/10/AGREE-II-Users-Manual-and-23-item-Instrument_2009_UPDATE_2013.pdf.
12. Richardson WS, Wilson MC, Nishikawa J, et al. The well-built clinical question: a key to evidence-based decisions. ACP J Club 1995;123:A12–3.
13. Guyatt GH, Oxman AD, Vist G, et al, for the GRADE Working Group. Rating quality of evidence and strength of recommendations GRADE: an emerging consensus on rating quality of evidence and strength of recommendations. BMJ 2008;336(7650):924–66.
14. Preferred practice guidelines: dry eye. American Academy of Ophthalmology; 2012. Available at: http://one.aao.org/summary-benchmark-detail/summary-benchmarks-complete-set-october-2012. Accessed August 19, 2014.
15. Christensen LB, Petersen PE, Thorn JJ, et al. Dental caries and dental health behavior of patients with primary Sjögren syndrome. Acta Odontol Scand 2001; 59(3):116–20.
16. Zero DT, Brennan MT, Daniels TE, et al. Clinical practice guidelines for oral management of Sjögren disease: Dental caries prevention. J Am Dent Assoc 2016; 147(4):295–305.
17. Quality of life impact of Sjögren's syndrome. The Moisture Seekers 2006;24:1–3.
18. Sjögren's syndrome foundation breakthrough goal survey. Polaris Marketing Research, Inc; 2012.
19. Mertzanis P, Abetz L, Rajagopalan K, et al. The relative burden of dry eye in patients' lives: comparisons to a U.S. normative sample. Invest Ophthalmol Vis Sci 2005;46:46–50.
20. Schiffman RM, Walt JG, Jacobsen G, et al. Utility assessment among patients with dry eye disease. Ophthalmology 2003;110:1412–9.

21. The definition and classification of dry eye disease: report of the Definition and Classification Subcommittee of the International Dry Eye Workshop (2007). Ocul Surf 2007;5:75–92.

22. Sullivan BD, Crews LA, Messmer EM, et al. Correlations between commonly used objective signs and symptoms for the diagnosis of dry eye disease: clinical implications. Acta Ophthalmol 2014;92:161–6.

23. Foulks GN, Forstot SL, Donshik PC, et al. Clinical Guidelines for Management of Dry Eye Associated with Sjögren Disease. Ocul Surf 2015;13(2):118–32.

24. Smedby KE, Vajdic CM, Falster M, et al. Autoimmune disorders and risk of non-Hodgkin lymphoma subtypes: a pooled analysis within the InterLymph Consortium. Blood 2008;111(8):4029–38.

25. Carsons SE, Parke A, Vivino FB, et al. Treatment guidelines for rheumatologic and systemic manifestations of Sjögren's: Use of biologics, management of fatigue and inflammatory musculoskeletal pain. Arthritis Care Res, in press.

26. Gottenberg JE, Ravaud P, Puéchal X, et al. Effects of hydroxychloroquine on symptomatic improvement in primary Sjögren syndrome: the JOQUER randomized clinical trial. JAMA 2014;312(3):249–58.

27. Fox RI, Chan E, Benton L, et al. Treatment of primary Sjögren's syndrome with hydroxychloroquine. Am J Med 1988;85(4A):62–7.

28. Fox RI, Dixon R, Guarrassi V, et al. Treatment of primary Sjögren's syndrome with hydroxychloroquine: a retrospective, open label study. Lupus 1996;5(Suppl 1): S31–6.

29. Tishler M, Yaron I, Shirazi I, et al. Hydroxychloroquine treatment for primary Sjögren's syndrome: its effect on salivary and serum inflammatory markers. Ann Rheum Dis 1999;58(4):253–6.

30. Fauchais AL, Ouattara B, Gondran G, et al. Articular manifestations in primary Sjögren's syndrome: clinical significance and prognosis of 188 patients. Rheumatology (Oxford) 2010;49(6):1164–72.

31. Skopouli FN, Jagiello P, Tsifetaki N, et al. Methotrexate in primary Sjögren's syndrome. Clin Exp Rheumatol 1996;14(5):555.

32. van Woerkom JM, Kruize AA, Geenen R, et al. Safety and efficacy of leflunomide in primary Sjögren's syndrome: a phase II pilot study. Ann Rheum Dis 2007;66(8): 1026–32.

33. Khan O, Carsons S. Occurrence of rheumatoid arthritis requiring oral and/or biological disease-modifying antirheumatic drug therapy following a diagnosis of primary Sjögren syndrome. J Clin Rheumatol 2012;18(7):356–8.

34. Segal B. Fatigue in primary Sjögren's syndrome. In: Ramos-Casals M, editor. Sjögren's syndrome: diagnosis and therapeutics. London: Springer Verlag; 2012. p. 129–43.

35. Strombeck BE, Theander E, Jacobsson LT. Effectiveness of exercise on aerobic capacity and fatigue in women with Primary Sjögren's syndrome. Rheumatology (Oxford) 2007;46(5):868–71.

36. Virkki LM, Porola P, Forsblad-d'Elia H, et al. Dehydroepiandrosterone (DHEA) substitution treatment for severe fatigue in DHEA-deficient patients with primary Sjögren's syndrome. Arthritis Care Res (Hoboken) 2010;62(1):118–24.

37. Hartkamp A, Geenen R, Godaert GL, et al. Effect of dehydroepiandrosterone administration on fatigue, well-being, and functioning in women with primary Sjögren syndrome: a randomised controlled trial. Ann Rheum Dis 2008;67(1): 91–7.

38. Sankar V, Brennan MT, Kok MR, et al. Etanercept in Sjögren's syndrome: a twelve-week randomized, double-blind, placebo-controlled pilot clinical trial. Arthritis Rheum 2004;50(7):2240–538.
39. Mariette X, Ravaud P, Steinfeld S, et al. Inefficacy of infliximab in primary Sjögren's syndrome: results of the randomized, controlled Trial of Remicade in Primary Sjögren's Syndrome (TRIPSS). Arthritis Rheum 2004;50(4):1270–6.
40. Devauchelle-Pensec V, Mariette X, Jousse-Joulin S, et al. Treatment of primary Sjögren syndrome with rituximab: a randomized trial. Ann Intern Med 2014; 160(4):233–42.
41. Faustman DL, Vivino FB, Carsons SE. Treatment of primary Sjögren's syndrome with rituximab: Comment on Devauchelle et al 2014. Ann Intern Med 2014; 161(5):376–7.
42. Meijer JM, Meiners PM, Vissink A, et al. Effectiveness of rituximab treatment in primary Sjögren's syndrome: a randomized, double-blind, placebo-controlled trial. Arthritis Rheum 2010;62(4):960–8.
43. Carubbi F, Cipriani P, Marrelli A, et al. Efficacy and safety of rituximab treatment in early primary Sjögren's syndrome: a prospective, multi-center, follow-up study. Arthritis Res Ther 2013;15(5):R172.
44. Pijpe J, van Imhoff GW, Vissink A, et al. Rituximab treatment in patients with primary Sjögren's syndrome: an open-label phase II study. Arthritis Rheum 2005; 52(9):2740–50.
45. Seror R, Sordet C, Guillevin L, et al. Tolerance and efficacy of rituximab and changes in serum B cell biomarkers in patients with systemic complications of primary Sjögren's syndrome. Ann Rheum Dis 2007;66(3):351–7.
46. Gorson KC, Natarajan N, Ropper AH, et al. Rituximab treatment in patients with IVIg-dependent immune polyneuropathy: a prospective pilot trial. Muscle Nerve 2007;35(1):66–9.
47. Gottenberg JE, Guillevin L, Lambotte O, et al. Club Rheumatismes et Inflammation (CRI). Tolerance and short term efficacy of rituximab in 43 patients with systemic autoimmune diseases. Ann Rheum Dis 2005;64(6):913–20.

Index

Note: Page numbers of article titles are in **boldface**.

A

Abatacept, 412, 414
Acetylcholine receptors, 424–425
AIR (Autoimmunité Rituximab) registry, 409
American-European Consensus Group, 458–459, 502
AMG 557/MED1587, 412
Anakinra, 410–411
Antibodies, **419–434**. *See also specific antigens,*.
Antimicrobials, for oral dryness, 537
ASAP studies, 414
Autoantibodies, **419–434**
Autoimmune epithelitis, 458
Autoimmune thyroid disease, 459, 461–463, 466
Autoimmunité Rituximab (AIR) registry, 409
Azathioprine, 542, 545

B

B cell(s)
 aggregation of, 476–478
 T-cell interaction with, 477
 therapy targeted to, 408–411
B lymphocyte tyrosine kinase, 439
Baminercept, 410, 413
B-cell activating factor, 474–475
B-cell activator of the TNF family, 408
 inhibitors of, 411
B-cell targets, for Sjögren's syndrome therapy, 408–411
Belimumab, 411–412
BELISS (Efficacy and Safety of Belimumab in Subjects with Primary Sjögren's
 Syndrome), 411
Biologics, **407–417,** 545–546
Biomarkers, in saliva, 451–453
Biopsy
 minor salivary glands, 486–487, 492–494
 parotid gland, **485–499**
B-lymphocyte chemoattractant, 439
Bronchiectasis, 422
Bruton tyrosine kinase, 413

Rheum Dis Clin N Am 42 (2016) 553–559
http://dx.doi.org/10.1016/S0889-857X(16)30034-5
0889-857X/16/$ – see front matter

Printed and bound by CPI Group (UK) Ltd, Croydon, CR0 4YY

08/05/2025

01864686-0005